D0784032

The Primary Care Guide to Mental Health

The Primary Care Guide to Mental Health

Sheila Hardy and Richard Gray

Primary Care Guide to Mental Health
Sheila Hardy
Richard Gray

ISBN: 978-1-905539-10-9

First published 2012

British Library Cataloguing in Publication Data

A catalogue record for this book is available from the British Library

Notice

Clinical practice and medical knowledge constantly evolve. Standard safety precautions must be followed, but, as knowledge is broadened by research, changes in practice, treatment and drug therapy may become necessary or appropriate. Readers must check the most current product information provided by the manufacturer of each drug to be administered and verify the dosages and correct administration, as well as contraindications. It is the responsibility of the practitioner, utilising the experience and knowledge of the patient, to determine dosages and the best treatment for each individual patient. Any brands mentioned in this book are as examples only and are not endorsed by the publisher. Neither the publisher nor the authors assume any liability for any injury and/or damage to persons or property arising from this publication.

To contact M&K Publishing write to:

M&K Update Ltd · The Old Bakery · St. John's Street

Keswick · Cumbria CA12 5AS

Tel: 01768 773030 · Fax: 01768 781099

publishing@mkupdate.co.uk

www.mkupdate.co.uk

Designed and typeset by Mary Blood
Printed in England by Ferguson Print, Keswick

For William John Patrick and Melita

Contents

List of tables

Foreword

One in three or four patients seen in primary care has a mental health problem. There are straightforward and effective treatments available for many of these conditions and some can be treated successfully by the primary healthcare clinicians themselves.

Many secondary care services for mental health are working towards earlier discharge, making primary care an important place for delivering mental healthcare. This has been recognised in the Quality and Outcomes Framework, giving clinicians in primary care responsibility for recognising and treating a certain number of mental illnesses. Clinicians in primary care need to work closely with those in mental health services to ensure the patient receives the most appropriate treatment.

This book aims to provide a straighforward guide to the mental health problems that are routinely managed in primary care. It is suitable for students and for clinicians working in primary care.

Glossary of terms

Agranulocytosis – decrease in the number of granulocytes in the blood

Antidepressant – medication used to treat anxiety and depression

Cardiovascular – relating to the heart and blood vessels

Cognitive – information-processing, including perception, learning, remembering, judging, and problem-solving

Co-morbid – the presence of one or more disorders

Congruent – the state of agreement

Delusion – a mistaken belief

Endocrine – relating to ductless glands

Galactorrhoea – spontaneous flow of milk from the breast

Gastrointestinal – relating to the stomach and intestine

Gynaecomastia – development of mammary glands in males

Hallucination – perceptions in the absence of external stimuli

Hyperprolactinaemia – abnormally high levels of prolactin in the blood

Leukopenia – a decrease in the number of white blood cells

Libido – desire for sexual activity

Locomotor – movement

Mania – a state of abnormally elevated or irritable mood, arousal, and/or energy levels

Micturition – ejection of urine from the bladder

Neurological – relating to the nervous system

Neutropenia – an abnormally low number of neutrophils in the blood

Palpitations – an abnormality of heartbeat that causes a conscious awareness of its beating

Pharmacological – the interaction between the body and the medication

Phobia – fear of an object or situation

Psychological – relating to the mind or emotions

Psychomotor retardation – slowing down of thought and a reduction of physical movements

Psychosis – loss of contact with reality

Schizoaffective – elevated and/or depressed mood, that alternates with, or occurs together with, distortions in perception

Abbreviations

APA – American Psychiatric Association

BMI – Body Mass Index

BPSD – Behavioural and Psychological Symptoms in Dementia

CBT – Cognitive Behavioural Therapy

CCBT – Computerised CBT

CHD – Coronary Heart Disease

COPD – Chronic Obstructive Pulmonary Disease

CPA – Care Programme Approach

CVD – Cardiovascular Disease

ECG – Electrocardiogram

EPS – Extrapyramidal Symptoms

IAPT – Improving Access to Psychological Therapy

IPT – Interpersonal Therapy

MUS – Medically Unexplained Symptoms

NaSSA – Noradrenergic and Specific Serotonergic Antidepressant

NMS – Neuroleptic Malignant Syndrome

OCD – Obsessive Compulsive Disorder

SESCAM – Side Effect Scale/Checklist for Antipsychotic Medication

SMI – Severe Mental Illness

SSRI – Selective Serotonin Reuptake Inhibitor

TCA – Tricyclic Antidepressant

TD – Tardive Dyskinesia

WRAP – Wellness Recovery Action Plan

Introduction

The Primary Care Team includes GPs, practice nurses, district nurses and health visitors. Some practices may employ their own counsellors. Access to other psychological therapies is still variable across the United Kingdom. When a patient presents to a member of this team with a mental health problem, they are assessed to see who will be the most appropriate person to manage their care. For most, this will be one of the people in the team and/or a primary care mental health professional. For patients who are suicidal or who have severe illness, referral to secondary care services is necessary.

Secondary care services are comprised of care in hospital or by the Community Mental Health Team (CMHT). The team includes psychiatrists, nurses, occupational therapists, clinical psychologists, social workers and support workers. After the CMHT have assessed any patient referred to them, they will send the GP a letter to inform them about their treatment and progress. The GP will then prescribe the medications recommended by the psychiatrist. Unless the patient is admitted to hospital, the GP remains responsible for the rest of the patient's medical care. If the patient is admitted to hospital, the GP will be kept informed of their progress and the discharge plan. When the patient is in hospital, the psychiatrist is responsible for their medical care. Families and friends, self-help and community groups also provide vital support to people with mental illness. Understanding and respecting each other's contribution enables conformity in who will provide which service to whom.

Chapter 1

Recovery

We are sure you have heard colleagues and patients talking about 'recovery' when discussing mental illness. The term has been popularised over the past decade and many mental health services promote themselves as being 'recovery focused'. For colleagues who work in primary care with patients who have both mental and physical disorders, talk about recovery may be a little confusing if not perplexing. It will be helpful, therefore, to discuss what is meant by recovery within a mental health context and how you as a primary care worker can support this approach.

Many mental health practitioners perceive that the functioning and quality of life of patients with severe mental illness (SMI) will inevitably decline over the course of the illness. Patients, it is argued, do not recover from SMI. Objectively there is a certain truth to this; psychosis is toxic and the longer people spend experiencing symptoms (for example, hearing voices, feeling paranoid, manic or depressed) the worse their functional outcomes. But this misses the point about how the concept of recovery is used in mental health. You may be thinking if a patient has a bout of influenza, they have recovered when the virus has run its course and the patient has returned to normal life. Patient groups have argued that recovery in mental health is different. Mental illness does not go away; to recover patients have to learn to work around or live with the symptoms they are experiencing. So much as you might like to help a patient with diabetes live with their condition (although you probably would not say they had recovered), by helping a patient with SMI work around their symptoms you may have helped to promote their recovery. This leads us to our second key observation about recovery; it is considered an ongoing process, not an outcome. So you can never say that a patient has recovered from mental illness; rather you have supported them in the process.

The concept of recovery in psychiatry emerged from patients writing about their experiences of living with mental illness in the early 1980s. Most famously

Pat Deegan (1988) talked about how she had developed skills in coping with her experiences, but perhaps most importantly about how to regain an identity beyond mental illness.

So in a mental health context you should consider recovery a process, an attitude, a guiding principle if you like. You may want to take some time to reflect on how comfortable this construct feels to you. Certainly there are many authors who have been very critical of the recovery concept and movement, lambasting it as no more than a marketing term used by mental health services to promote themselves. We consider that the message of hope and positive collaboration that the recovery concept imbues is an important consideration for professionals, patients and their carers.

How do I promote recovery?

Using a recovery approach places an increasing emphasis on self-management and a strengths approach, focusing on what people can do, rather than what they can't, and looking at social, as opposed to medical, outcomes. Housing, employment, education and participation in mainstream community and leisure activities become the central objectives.

Geoff Shepherd (Shepherd *et al.*, 2008) offers us ten top tips for recovery oriented practice. He suggests that after each consultation, you should ask yourself, did I...

1. actively listen to help the person to make sense of their mental health problems?
2. help the person identify and prioritise their personal goals for recovery, not professional goals?
3. demonstrate a belief in the person's existing strengths and resources in relation to the pursuit of these goals?
4. identify examples from my own lived experience, or that of other patients, which inspire and validate their hopes?
5. pay particular attention to the importance of goals which take the person out of the 'sick role' and enable them actively to contribute to the lives of others?
6. identify non-mental health resources – friends, contacts, organisations – relevant to the achievement of their goals?
7. encourage self-management of mental health problems (by providing information, reinforcing existing coping strategies, etc.)?

8. discuss what the person wants in terms of therapeutic interventions, e.g. psychological treatments, alternative therapies, joint crisis planning, etc., respecting their wishes wherever possible?

9. behave at all times so as to convey an attitude of respect for the person and a desire for an equal partnership in working together, indicating a willingness to 'go the extra mile'?

10. while accepting that the future is uncertain and setbacks will happen, continue to express support for the possibility of achieving these self-defined goals, maintaining hope and positive expectations?

These tips are helpful in guiding our overall practice towards a more recovery oriented approach to working with people with mental health problems. Other authors have described different stages of recovery. Knowing which stage in the recovery process your patient has reached, will enable you to target your interventions more effectively. Table 1.1 shows Andresen and colleagues' (2006) five stage model of recovery. To work out which recovery stage your patient is at, you can use the Stages of Recovery Instrument (STORI) also developed by Andresen *et al.* (2006). The STORI is a fifty item self-report measure; each item is rated on a five point scale. You can find out more about this measure by going to the following website: http://www.uow.edu.au/health/iimh/stori/index.html (last accessed: 24.4.11).

Table 1.1 *Five stages of recovery*

1. Moratorium	A time of withdrawal characterised by a profound sense of loss and hopelessness
2. Awareness	Realisation that all is not lost and that a fulfilling life is possible
3. Preparation	Taking stock of strengths and weaknesses regarding recovery and starting to work on developing recovery skills
4. Rebuilding	Actively working towards a positive identity, setting meaningful goals and taking control of one's life
5. Growth	Living a meaningful life, characterised by self-management of the illness, resilience and a positive sense of self

Source: Andresen *et al.* (2006).

At each of the five stages it has been argued that different therapeutic techniques may be particularly helpful. We have listed some below under the five stage subheadings.

Moratorium

At this stage, the professional:

- demonstrates hope and the potential for achievement when interacting with the patient;
- promotes acceptance as first step to recovery;
- explains illness, symptoms/distressing experiences, courses of treatment;
- informs the patient about benefits of active treatment;
- engages family and/or significant others and refers them to available community supports and education.

Awareness

At this stage, the professional:

- ensures the patient and family/significant others are educated about the choices/resources available to them;
- provides activities that will increase the patient's readiness to make choices in selecting life roles, environment, and goals;
- educates the patient about mental illness and recovery;
- continues to use hope-inspiring strategies.

Preparation and Rebuilding

At this stage, the professional:

- assists the person in connecting with ordinary community services based upon their needs;
- works with the person to review and monitor status of their goals;
- assists the person in contacting agencies and services that will help them achieve life goals and support recovery-enhancing activities (i.e. recovery groups, housing options, volunteer opportunities);
- refers to employment agencies to learn about how to use work incentives;
- supports and assists the person in developing personal coping skills.

Growth

At this stage, the professional:

- provides support/assistance in maintaining recovery;
- advocates use of community resources;
- encourages and supports the person in becoming more involved in community activities;

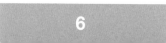

- keeps patients/family/significant others up-to-date about new medications, alternatives and complementary treatments.

Having set out some fairly general therapeutic techniques for promoting recovery, it might now be helpful to focus on Wellness Recovery Action Planning, a specific clinical tool that is increasingly used by mental health practitioners working within a recovery framework.

Wellness Recovery Action Planning (WRAP)

Mary Ellen Copeland has personal experience of mental illness that she has used in developing the WRAP. The philosophy that underpins the WRAP is that prevention is better than cure. The WRAP is an individualised workbook that aims to enable the patient to take control over the problems or difficulties they experience in their day-to-day lives. There is no particular way in which the workbook has to be completed. Some WRAPs are short and sweet, some contain pictures, and others are detailed personal accounts of lived experiences. Patients can work on their WRAP on their own; many, however, say that they find it valuable to have someone they trust to work on it with them. The thoughts and reflections that patients have written in their WRAP serve to remind and guide and also as a resource and source of comfort when times are difficult. Each WRAP will be individual and unique but in our experience we usually find included:

1. Taking each day at a time – the patient will identify what they are like when they are well and what they do to keep feeling well. They will also identify some of the things they may wish to work on to keep themselves well.

2. Understanding triggers – the patient will explore their personal triggers and consider what they can do to avoid and control them.

3. Identifying warning signs – early warning signs are the subtle signs of changes in the patient's thoughts or feelings or behaviour, which indicate that they may need to take action to avoid a worsening of their condition or situation.

4. Supporters – the patient will list the people who could provide some additional support when things get difficult. They can be family members, work colleagues, friends or healthcare professionals.

You can find out a lot more about WRAPs by visiting the following website: http://www.mentalhealthrecovery.com/ (last accessed: 2.1.12).

Summary

Recovery is a process not a goal. In this chapter we have considered how you as a primary care practitioner can work within a recovery framework in your consultations with patients. At the core of the recovery approach to working with patients with mental health problems is the fostering of hope. We have discussed the Stages of Recovery Instrument as a tool to identify which stage of recovery the patient is in to guide more focused intervention, and Wellness Recovery Action Plans to help patients develop their own strategies for managing their lives.

Case Study

Mary is 36 years old. She was in an abusive relationship and consequently became very depressed and anxious. She did have a responsible office job but has been unable to work for the last two years due to the severity of her anxiety symptoms. Mary has been treated with antidepressant medication and has had support from her family and the practice nurse. Mary's hope is to go back to work and feel part of a team again. She has expressed a tentative readiness to prepare for this.

The practice nurse identified an organisation which encourages people to volunteer with them, doing the type of work they are good at. She explained that Mary would be able to take a member of her family to the interview with her and start by working just a few hours. Mary said that this made her feel much less anxious. Together they worked out a plan of the steps Mary would need to take in order to organise the interview.

References

Andresen, R., Caputi, P. and Oades, L. (2006) Stages of recovery instrument: development of a measure of recovery from serious mental illness. *Australian and New Zealand Journal of Psychiatry* **40**: 972–80.

Deegan, P. (1988) Recovery: The lived experience of rehabilitation. *Psychiatric Rehabilitation Journal* **11**: 11–19.

Shepherd, G., Boardman, J. and Slade, M. (2008) *Making Recovery a Reality.* London: Sainsbury Centre for Mental Health.

Chapter 2

Depression

Most people with depression will be managed in primary care. In this chapter we will consider how to identify depression and review the treatments which you as primary care clinicians can offer. Everybody's mood fluctuates over time; much of the time people will describe themselves as feeling ok (euthymic). In response to a range of biological, psychological and social (biopsychosocial) factors our mood may be negatively affected. People often, therefore, will talk about their mood as being down or flat. This is not depression. Only when people experience low mood for a prolonged period of time do we start to consider that they might be experiencing a depressive illness. Depression severity can range from mild, through moderate to severe, and commonly co-exists with other long-term health problems. So in primary care the presenting complaint may be listed as somatic (physical) when in fact the real problem is depression.

Depression is often a response to biopsychosocial (life) events that typically include relationship or financial problems, physical illness, bereavement, moving house or redundancy. Some people, however, can become depressed for no obvious reason and it is important to remember that their suffering is just as real as those who are reacting to events that have occurred. Characterised by loss of hope, not being able to think clearly, lethargy, sleep problems, changes in appetite and irritability, you should think about depression as a constellation of symptoms, not simply an illness characterised by low mood.

Epidemiology

The World Health Organization (WHO, 2004) projections suggest that by 2030, depression will be the leading cause of disease burden in developed countries. It is a very common illness; about two-thirds of adults will at some time experience some degree of depressed mood sufficient to negatively impact on their day-to-day lives

(Stewart *et al.*, 2004). Each year six per cent of the adult population will develop a depressive illness.

Of every one hundred people you see in primary care between five and ten will be suffering from a depressive disorder (Katon and Schulberg, 1992), making it the third most common reason for attendance. So if you see 40 patients in a day you should expect between two and four of them to have depression.

Mild and moderate depression are the most common forms of the illness with respectively, a lifetime prevalence of 17 and 6 per cent. Severe depression is much less common with fewer than 3 per cent suffering from this form of the illness.

Let us now consider the symptoms of depression and how to make a diagnosis.

Symptoms of depression

Our experience working in primary care is that our patients may typically present complaining of physical symptoms. Alternatively they are persuaded to come in by a close family member who has noticed they are not eating, sleeping, are more irritable, have lost interest in sex and may say 'my wife told me to come and see you because…'. In no particular order these are the common physical and psychological depression symptoms you will find in patients that come and see you. Patients may experience few or many of these symptoms to a greater or lesser severity.

Physical symptoms

- Change in appetite: not eating resulting in weight loss, eating excessively resulting in weight gain, unhealthy eating resulting in poorer physical wellbeing.
- Bowel changes: constipation, diarrhoea or preoccupation with bowel function.
- Participation in daily life: the patient lacks vitality and may sit and brood. Everyday tasks such as washing and dressing may be difficult to perform. Generally the patient's actions are slowed down.
- General appearance: sad and miserable, often unkempt (or badly dressed).
- Sexual function: partial or total loss of libido (sex drive). Amenorrhoea (partial or complete stopping of periods) may be experienced by some women.

- Sleep disturbance: difficulty in getting to sleep. The sleep may be broken with excessive dreaming; the patient wakes up unrefreshed and then feels tired and unable to get going in the morning. Some people wake up two or three hours before usual waking time and do not get back to sleep.
- Other physical symptoms: dry mouth, indigestion, palpitations, headaches, giddiness, tight band round chest and head, skin-picking, hand-wringing, general aches and pains.

Psychological symptoms
- Depressed mood: feelings of sadness, feeling low or flat.
- Attitude: feeling fed up, indecisive, preoccupation with physical symptoms, indifference, denial or lack of awareness of symptoms.
- Loss of interest in life: withdrawal from the outside world, reduced awareness of current events, lacking interest in what is going on around them.
- Speech: slow, monotonous, monosyllabic answers. Incessant negative talk, often about death, dying and the futility of life.
- Thought: slow and difficult, poor concentration, preoccupation with morbid thoughts (death/suicide).

It is worth screening all patients who attend primary care for depression. This need take no more than a few minutes. We know that patients who are depressed frequently consult primary care on several occasions, often with physical problems, before the depression is picked up. So it is worth you investing time in screening patients for depression because if it is identified and treated, patients with depression will be considerably less burdensome to the practice (and of course be healthier).

Screening for depression
We strongly recommend that you screen every patient you see every time you see them for depression. Remember statistically two to four patients you see every day are depressed. You should pay particular attention to screening patients in key high risk groups. They are:
- patients with significant physical illness, e.g. diabetes, cardiovascular disease, COPD, stroke;
- patients with other mental health problems, such as dementia;

- patients suffering due to major life events;
- patients with a history of relationship difficulties and physical, sexual or emotional abuse.

How do I possibly screen every patient?

You can screen patients for depression by asking two simple questions, the so called Whooley or two question test. Patients simply answer 'yes' or 'no'; if they answer yes to either question you should explore whether this is something they want help with and consider further assessment of the mood symptoms they are experiencing. The questions are:

1. 'During the last month have you often been bothered by feeling down, depressed, or hopeless?'

2. 'During the last month have you often been bothered by having little interest or pleasure in doing things?'

Some primary care practitioners argue that the use of these standardised questions is unnecessary. If they are not used, up to seven out of ten cases of depression will go undetected (Arroll *et al.*, 2005). We therefore strongly recommend their routine use.

If depression is suspected, either clinically or from the results of the screening questions, you should assess for the level of depression using an assessment tool validated for use in primary care. Most patients are quite willing to complete these assessments if they are introduced sensitively with a clear explanation of the reason you have asked them to do it. For example:

'Would you please fill out this form? It will only take a few minutes. It will help us understand more about how you have been feeling, and how we can both make decisions to help you to move forward.'

The Patient Health Questionnaire (PHQ-9) is perhaps the mostly widely used depression screening tool and is available for use free of charge without permission from:

http://www.phqscreeners.com/terms.aspx (last accessed 2.1.12).

The PHQ-9 scores each of the nine DSM-IV criteria on a zero (not at all) to three (nearly every day) scale. Scores of five, ten, fifteen and twenty represent cut-off points for mild, moderate, moderately severe and severe depression respectively. A total score greater than or equal to ten has 88 per cent sensitivity and specificity for major depression. It should be noted, however that after assessing the relative validity of the PHQ-9, HADS-D, and the World Health Organization Well-Being Index against the Structured Clinical Interview for DSM-IV (SCID), Lowe *et al.* (2004) recommend a cut-off point of ≥11 for major depression for the PHQ-9.

Diagnosis

The Diagnostic and Statistical Manual of Mental Disorders (4th Edition; DSM-IV, APA (2000)) criteria are recommended for health professionals in the United Kingdom to use in making a diagnosis of a (major) depressive episode (a one-off event) or disorder (long-term condition). We summarise the criteria here:

- To meet the criteria for a major depressive episode the patients should have been experiencing at least five of the following symptoms for at least two weeks; at least one of the symptoms must be depressed mood or loss of interest or pleasure. Your diagnosis will be based on what the patient or family member tells you and what you observe during your consultation:

  1. Depressed mood most of the day, nearly every day (e.g. feels sad or empty).

  2. Markedly diminished interest or pleasure in all, or almost all, activities most of the day, nearly every day (anhedonia).

  3. Significant weight loss when not dieting or weight gain (e.g., a change of more than 5 per cent of body weight in a month), or decrease or increase in appetite nearly every day.

  4. Insomnia or hypersomnia nearly every day.

  5. Psychomotor agitation or retardation nearly every day.

  6. Fatigue or loss of energy nearly every day.

  7. Feelings of worthlessness or excessive or inappropriate guilt (which may be delusional) nearly every day (not merely self-reproach or guilt about being sick).

  8. Diminished ability to think or concentrate, or indecisiveness, nearly every day.

  9. Recurrent thoughts of death (not just fear of dying), recurrent suicidal ideation without a specific plan, or a suicide attempt or a specific plan for committing suicide.

- To make a diagnosis of depression the symptoms must also cause distress or impairment in social or occupational functioning.

- You would not make a diagnosis of major depression if the symptoms
  - meet the criteria for a mixed episode (i.e. anxiety and depression)
  - are associated with the physiological effects of a substance (e.g. a drug of abuse, a medication), or a medical condition (e.g. hypothyroidism).
  - are better accounted for by bereavement or psychosis.
- You would also not make a diagnosis of major depression if there has ever been a manic, mixed (mania and depression) or hypomanic episode.

If the symptoms that presented during your consultation with the patient have been present for more than two months you should consider whether the patient meets the criteria for a major depressive disorder rather than a single episode.

Risk assessment

It is a sad fact that 1 in 30 patients with depression will attempt suicide and 1 in 300 will be successful in killing themselves. Good risk assessment is therefore an essential part of the care and management of patients with depression. It is important that you directly ask depressed patients about current suicidal ideas and intent and ask if they feel hopeless or that life is not worth living. A family history of suicide and past attempts are significant risk factors; consequently as part of a comprehensive risk assessment, it is important that you also ask detailed questions about both of these. If suicidal ideation is present, it is essential to determine whether the patient has a current suicide plan and their resolve to carry out the plan.

If a patient does have suicidal ideas, you will need to measure whether they have adequate social support and are aware of sources of help. Patients with depression and their carers need to be vigilant for changes in mood, negativity and hopelessness, and suicidal intent, particularly during high-risk periods (such as initiation of, or changes to antidepressant medication, or at times of increased stress). You should advise them to contact an appropriate healthcare professional if they are concerned or if their situation deteriorates.

The following questions will be helpful to use in assessing patients:
- Earlier attempt – Have you made a suicide attempt in the past?
- Thoughts – Do you think that life is not worth living?

Do you think about harming or killing yourself?
- Plan – Have you got a plan to kill yourself? How would you do it?
- Aim – Do you aim to carry out this plan?

- Tools – Have you got access to (the necessary tools to) carry out the plan? For example: a supply of medication if planning an overdose.
- Stop – What would stop (or what is stopping) you from carrying out your plan? For example: they wouldn't want to abandon their children.

Disclaimer: The advice we have given is intended to inform and guide clinical practice around the detection and prevention of suicide risk. Practitioners are, at all times, responsible for their own practice. If you are not able to demonstrate competence in undertaking a risk assessment you must, as a matter of urgency, refer to a colleague who can.

Treatment of depression in Primary Care

Mild depression

For people with mild depression (i.e. those with a PHQ-9 score ≤5) you should consider the following treatments:
- Offer them the opportunity to talk about their problems without offering advice, judgement or possible solutions.
- Arrange a further assessment, normally within two weeks.
- Provide general information about depression and its treatments.
- Maintain contact with the patient to ensure their depression does not become more severe.

Moderate depression

For people with moderate depression (i.e. those with a PHQ-9 score of 6–10) you should, depending on patient preference, offer a choice of the following 'low-intensity' interventions:

Working to increase helpful behaviour (behavioural activation)
Encouraging patients to increase adaptive behaviours (such as exercise, socialising, working) has been shown to be useful in treating depression. This is often described as behavioural activation – doing activities that make you feel less depressed.

Computerised cognitive behavioural therapy (cCBT)
CCBT is a web based self help treatment. The four main packages are: Beating the Blues (which has to be installed on a computer terminal, often in the

surgery) (**http://www.beatingtheblues.co.uk** – last accessed: 2.1.12) Fear Fighter (**www.fearfighter.com** – last accessed: 2.1.12); Living Life to the Full (**www.livinglifetothefull.com** – last accessed 2.1.12) and Mood Gym (**www.moodgym.anu.edu.au** – last accessed 2.1.12). Whilst there is evidence that these interventions can be effective, there are issues with patients adhering to the intervention. They appear to be most effective with support from a primary care professional.

Structured group physical activity programme

Physical activity is an effective treatment for mild and moderate depression. You may, in your area, have a structured group programme available for patients. The programme is facilitated by a qualified instructor and typically consists of three sessions per week (lasting 45 minutes to one hour) over a 10 to 14 week period.

Moderate and severe depression

People with a moderate to severe depressive disorder (i.e. with a PHQ-9 score ≥15) will require treatment with either antidepressant medication (typically an SSRI such as fluoxetine and citalopram at standard doses), cognitive behavioural therapy (CBT), interpersonal therapy (IPT, helping patients solve the problems that are driving the depression), or a combination of medication and psychological treatments. In primary care CBT and IPT can be offered by IAPT professionals (Improving Access to Psychological Therapy). The choice of treatment should take into account patient preference.

Treatment refractory depression

Some patients with a moderate to severe depression fail to respond to treatment and are sometimes referred to as treatment refractory. If patients don't respond to CBT or IPT, then you should give them an antidepressant. For patients treated with antidepressants who have failed to respond to an adequate dose given for an adequate duration (e.g. 20mg/day of fluoxetine for two months), then you should switch them to a different drug.

Postnatal Depression (PND)

Depression affects 10–15% of women postnatally. Onset usually starts within one or two months of giving birth but can be later. In approximately one-third of women, symptoms start in pregnancy. Not be confused with the baby blues (which over half of new mothers will experience three to ten days following birth)

PND is a mental disorder that requires intervention.

Women are more likely to have PND if they:

- have a history of mental health problems
- suffered a recent traumatic event or are under stress
- experienced depression or anxiety during pregnancy
- have little support from either family or friends.

The Edinburgh Post Natal Depression Scale (EPNDS) should be offered to women as an essential part of routine care in the postnatal period (you can download it from:

http://www.fresno.ucsf.edu/pediatrics/downloads/edinburghscale.pdf (last accessed 2.1.12). When patients attend primary care, it is worth taking the oppportunity to screen them for depression using EPNDS. Diagnosis and treatment of PND should follow guidelines for unipolar depression used in the general population (either psychological or antidepressant treatment). There is evidence, however, that in breastfeeding women treated with antidepressants, the drug is found in the mother's milk. Psychological treatments may therefore be a logical first choice treatment for women with PND.

Postpartum (Puerperal) psychosis

Postpartum (Puerperal) psychosis affects 1 in 1000 women. It can develop within a few hours, days or weeks after childbirth. Symptoms may include rapid mood swings, delusions or hallucinations. Urgent referral to secondary care is essential to ensure effective treatment is initiated.

Review and offer referral from primary care
If after trying several different depression treatments and the patient remains depressed then referral to specialist mental health services may be appropriate. It should be noted, however, that secondary mental health services are often reticent to accept referrals of patients with depression.

Summary

Recognition and diagnosis is the pivotal first step to ensuring this group of patients are effectively treated. The vast majority of depressed patients can be effectively treated in primary care utilising a range of effective pharmacological and psychological treatments.

John is 65. He had just retired when his wife announced that she was leaving to live with another man. John was devastated. After a few weeks he decided to visit the GP because he could not sleep, was comfort eating, was unable to apply himself to any tasks, had no interest in the house or how he looked and felt 'awful'. The GP used the PHQ-9 tool to assess the severity of his condition which was moderate to severe. The risk assessment revealed that John had no thoughts of suicide. The GP suggested antidepressants, explained their effects and how long John should take them for. John agreed to take fluoxetine 20mg daily.

At his next appointment two weeks later John said he was starting to feel a little bit better. He still woke early in the morning and found it too difficult to do any jobs but was eating less and getting washed and dressed. The GP referred John to the IAPT worker who worked with John using behavioural activation.

References

American Psychiatric Association (APA) (2000) *Diagnostic and Statistical Manual of Mental Disorders (DSM)*. 4th edn. Arlington, VA: APA.

Arroll, B., Goodyear-Smith, F., Kerse, N., Fishman, T. and Gunn, J. (2005) Effect of the addition of a 'help' question to two screening questions on specificity for diagnosis of depression in general practice: diagnostic validity study. *British Medical Journal* **331**: 884.

Katon, W. and Schulberg, H. (1992) Epidemiology of depression in primary care. *General Hospital Psychiatry* **14** (4): 237–47.

Lowe, B., Spitzer, R.L., Grafe, K., Kroenke, K., Quenter, A,, Zipfel, S., Bucholz, C., Witte, S. and Herzog, W. (2004) Comparative validity of three screening questionnaires for DSM-IV depressive disorders and physicians' diagnoses. *Journal of Affective Disorders* **78**: 131–40.

Stewart, D., Gucciardi, E. and Grace, S. (2004) Depression. *BMC Women's Health* **25** (4) Suppl 1: S19.

World Health Organization (2004) *The Global Burden of Disease 2004 update*. Switzerland: WHO.

Chapter 3

Anxiety

Anxiety is a common mental disorder generally exclusively treated in primary care. In this chapter we will consider how to identify anxiety and review the treatments which you as primary care clinicians can offer.

Anxiety as a disorder is the extreme of a normal stress reaction: the fight or flight response. When faced with a stressful event (e.g. you are about to be eaten by a lion) your body adapts psychologically and physically, enabling you to either run away or fight to your maximum ability. In modern society (where there are few lions) this fight or flight response can be triggered in more inappropriate ways, for example, before a job interview, where the ability to run away quickly is not so helpful; this is not an anxiety disorder.

Anxiety disorders occur when the fight or flight response is prompted in certain circumstances. Examples might include: the thought of going out, meeting new people, seeing a picture of a spider in a book, leaving the house in a mess. So anxiety can therefore be considered a normal reaction to an inappropriate stimulus. Anxiety disorders can be disabling because people start to avoid things that make them anxious. So a person, whose fight or flight response is triggered by going out of the house, stops going out; the person who worries about their messy house, cleans constantly and doesn't ever invite friends round.

Epidemiology

In the United Kingdom approximately three per cent of people will develop anxiety during a given year, and at any one point in time around five per cent (300,000 people) of the population will have an anxiety disorder (ONS, 2000).

More women suffer from anxiety than men. Barlow (2001) tells us that there is a 2:1 female to male ratio for anxiety. Anxiety can affect people of all ages, though it is seen more widely in the elderly and less commonly in people aged between 15 and 24 years.

How does anxiety present in Primary Care?

Patients with anxiety disorders typically present in primary care with physical symptoms (a racing heart, bowel problems, rapid breathing) that are caused by their anxiety. Often these will be investigated and found to have no apparent cause (medically unexplained symptoms or MUS); it is of course important to investigate, in the first instance, any physical cause of these symptoms. Some patients with an anxiety disorder will present saying that they are feeling anxious, but in our experience, at least in Primary Care, this is unusual.

Typical physical complaints that patients with anxiety disorder present with include:

- cardiovascular symptoms such as palpitations, tachycardia, chest pain (I am having a heart attack), alteration in skin colour and abnormal blood pressure (both high or low);
- endocrine symptoms such as dry mouth;
- gastrointestinal symptoms that include nausea, vomiting, burping, constipation or diarrhoea, loss or increase in appetite, dry mouth and weight loss;
- locomotor symptoms including increased muscle tension and weakness, tremor, and akathisia (restlessness);
- reproductive symptoms such as decreased libido (men may experience erectile dysfunction) and increased menstrual flow;
- respiratory symptoms: panting for air, tightness of the chest, increased respirations, sweating, cold clammy palms, sighing;
- urinary symptoms including frequency of micturition, stress incontinence;
- other symptoms such as insomnia, blurred vision, headache, pins and needles in hands and feet, giddiness, tinnitus, preoccupation with ill-health.

Whilst it is important to check if there is a physical cause to these symptoms, you should be mindful that patients may seek additional tests or second opinions that are unnecessary and expensive. Even though the symptoms the patient is reporting may have no physical cause, it is still important to acknowledge the distress they may be experiencing and suggest that anxiety may be a possible cause.

What are the psychological symptoms of anxiety?

Alongside the physical symptoms we have outlined, patients may also experience

a wide range of psychological symptoms of anxiety, these include:
- poor concentration
- feelings of helplessness
- fatigue
- bizarre thoughts
- wanting to run away from a feared situation
- irritability and restlessness
- thoughts of insecurity and inferiority.

Different types of anxiety disorder

The most common anxiety disorders that you will see in Primary Care are:
- Panic disorder
  - Characterised by recurrent unexpected panic attacks.
- Phobias
  - Social phobia, marked out by a persistent fear of social or performance situations.
  - Agoraphobia, a dread of leaving the house, entering public places or travelling alone.
- OCD (obsessive compulsive disorder), defined by obsessions or compulsions (or both) for example repeated handwashing, checking the house is locked or plugs are turned off, the need for straightness.

Screening for anxiety

Screening for anxiety can be done quickly and simply by asking two key questions:

1. **'Do you feel nervous, anxious or on edge?' Yes/No**

2. **'Do you feel unable to stop worrying?' Yes/No**

These questions are sufficiently sensitive to detect the majority of patients who are anxious. Asking a third question will considerably improve specifity (i.e. will help you screen out people who don't actually have an anxiety disorder):

3. **'Is this something with which you would like help?' No/Yes, but not today/ Yes**

If anxiety is suspected, either clinically or from the results of the screening questions, you should assess further using a validated assessment measure for use in primary care (e.g. the GAD7). The Generalised Anxiety Disorder assessment

(GAD7) is an easy to use, self-administered patient questionnaire that can be used as a screening tool and severity measure for anxiety disorder (Swinson, 2006). The GAD7 can be downloaded from **http://www.phqscreeners.com/terms.aspx** (last accessed: 2.1.12) or is available as a computerised tool on Patient UK: **http://www. patient.co.uk/showdoc/40026141/** (last accessed: 2.1.12).

The phobia scale should be used together with the GAD7. It is available as a computerised tool on Patient UK: **http://www.patient.co.uk/doctor/IAPT-Phobia-Scale.htm** (last accessed: 2.1.12).

Most patients are quite willing to complete these assessments if they are introduced sensitively with a clear explanation of the reason you have asked them to do it.

Risk assessment

A study by Sareen *et al.* (2005) confirmed that having an anxiety disorder is an independent risk factor for suicide. In patients with an anxiety disorder you should assess for suicide risk using the questions described in the previous chapter.

Treatment of anxiety in Primary Care

There are a range of treatments available for treating anxiety, including medication and CBT.

Medication

There is evidence that high doses of selective serotonin reuptake inhibitors (SSRIs) can be effective in the treatment of anxiety disorders (e.g. 60mg/day of fluoxetine). Benzodiazepines can be helpful in the short-term management of anxiety disorder (no more than a two week course should be prescribed) but are NOT a long-term treatment option as dependency quickly develops. See Chapter 10 on medication.

Cognitive Behavioural Therapy (CBT)

There are decades of evidence that CBT is a highly effective treatment for anxiety disorders. Repeated exposure to the feared situation, making the patient as anxious as they can possibly endure, will, if patients adhere to the therapy, decrease the anxiety, enabling the patient to move on with their lives. CBT can be accessed in Primary Care through IAPT.

Summary

Many of the patients you see in Primary Care who have an anxiety disorder will typically present with physical problems. We have set out how to screen for anxiety in your patients. Anxiety disorders can be very effectively treated with CBT or medication.

Susan is 36 years old. She went to see her GP because she was worried about her heart which felt like it was going much too fast. She was also getting lots of headaches, stiffness in her arms and legs and feeling sick. The GP checked her blood pressure and pulse which were normal. On taking a history he discovered that Susan was under a lot of pressure at work and was struggling to complete her workload. He asked Susan the screening questions and she replied positively. The GAD7 test revealed that Susan was suffering from mild to moderate anxiety. Susan was relieved to learn that her physical symptoms could be caused by her anxiety. The GP advised Susan that medication was not indicated in her case and asked Susan if there was anyone she could talk to at work. Susan said her line manager was very good but she had not wanted to let her down. She now realised that she needed to go and talk to her. The GP made an appointment for Susan to see him in two weeks time.

References

Barlow, D.H. (ed.) (2001) *Clinical Handbook of Psychological Disorders* (3rd edn). New York: Guilford Press.

Office of National Statistics (ONS) (2000) *Psychiatric Morbidity among Adults living in Private Households.* London: Office of National Statistics.

Sareen, J., Cox, B., Afifi, T., de Graaf, R., Asmundson, G., ten Have, M. and Stein, M. (2005) *Anxiety Disorders and Risk for Suicidal Ideation and Suicide Attempts.* Retrieved 1 August 2010 from Archives of General Psychiatry website: http://archpsyc.ama-assn.org/cgi/content/full/62/11/1249 (last accessed: 24.4.11).

Swinson, R. (2006) The GAD-7 scale was accurate for diagnosing generalised anxiety disorder. *Evidence-Based Medicine* **11**(6): 184.

Chapter 4
Depression and Anxiety

Symptoms of depression and anxiety frequently co-exist so it is very common for people with depression to also experience anxiety and vice versa. Although the 'mixed depression and anxiety' label is commonly used in clinical practice it is not a recognised diagnostic code. A mixture of depression and anxiety symptoms is one of the most common reasons why patients attend primary care. Typically, patients may present with a low mood and other depression symptoms but will also experience considerable anxiety and/or worry. They may also talk about the physical rather than mental symptoms they are experiencing. These may include problems with sleeping, fatigue or loss of energy, poor concentration, disturbed appetite, dry mouth, tension and restlessness, tremor, palpitations, dizziness and loss of libido. We have already made this point but it is worth reiterating; both depression and anxiety are a mixture of both mental AND physical symptoms.

Epidemiology

In the UK the point prevalence (the percentage of the population actually with the condition) of mixed depression and anxiety among adults (i.e. those aged 16–74 years of age) in 2000 was 11 per cent (Singleton *et al.*, 2001). As with both depression and anxiety, as separate conditions, more women (14 per cent) than men (9 per cent) suffer from co-occurring depression and anxiety symptoms (Singleton *et al.*, 2001).

Compared to patients who have received a single diagnosis of either depression or anxiety those with co-occurring disorders are more likely to have worse psychosocial and treatment outcomes, poorer quality of life, are less likely to stick to treatment, recover more slowly, are more likely to kill themselves, and use health services more.

Screening for anxiety and depression

In Chapters 2 and 3 we respectively described screening questions for depression and anxiety. Because depression and anxiety so commonly co-exist we recommend, largely on pragmatic grounds, that every patient is screened for depression and anxiety using the following screening questions (this should take no more than about 30 seconds of your time per patient and is time well spent).

Depression screening questions (yes/no response)
1. During the last month have you often been bothered by feeling down, depressed, or hopeless?
2. During the last month have you often been bothered by having little interest or pleasure in doing things?

Anxiety screening questions (yes/no response)
1. Do you feel nervous, anxious or on edge?
2. Do you feel unable to stop worrying?

It has been found that the specificity (the percentage of healthy people who are correctly identified as not having the condition) of both of these two question tests is improved if you ask the following supplementary question and only further assess patients that give a 'yes, but not today' or 'yes' response (ruling out people who answer 'yes' to both questions but are not actually depressed or anxious).

Supplementary question (no/yes, but not today/yes response)
'Is this something with which you would like help?'

Assessment of depression and anxiety symptoms

We have described in some detail in Chapters 2 and 3 respectively the standardised measures for depression and anxiety symptoms. These include (for depression) the PHQ-9, (for anxiety) the GAD7 and phobia scale. Some colleagues use in practice the Hospital Anxiety and Depression scale (HAD; Zigmond and Snaith, 1983). The HAD is a self-report screening questionnaire for depression and anxiety. The major benefit of the HAD over the other assessment tools we have described is that it addresses both depression and anxiety and gives separate scores for both. Perhaps because of copyright restrictions the HAD is becoming less popular in practice (although it remains a popular research instrument).

Diagnosis

We have summarised the American Psychiatric Association (APA) diagnostic criteria for anxiety and depression in Chapters 2 and 3 (APA ,2000). It is interesting to note that the APA has proposed diagnostic criteria for mixed anxiety and depression (APA, 2010). They are that the patient has three or four of the symptoms of major depression (see Chapter 2) which must include depressed mood and/or anhedonia and be accompanied by anxious distress (having two or more of the following symptoms: irrational worry, preoccupation with unpleasant worries, having trouble relaxing, motor tension, fear that something awful may happen). The symptoms must have lasted at least two weeks, and no other DSM diagnosis of anxiety or depression must be present; they must both be occurring at the same time.

Risk Assessment

A risk assessment should be carried out as described in Chapter 2.

Treatment of mixed depression and anxiety

If a patient has co-occurring depression and anxiety there is a simple rule that you should always follow. Treat the depression first and the anxiety will take care of itself. If the patient presents with an anxiety disorder (such as OCD or Phobia) rather than symptoms and it is this disorder that is driving the depression then (and there is no hard and fast rule about this) it may be worth considering treating the anxiety first. Most patients with persistent and/or severe symptoms of anxiety and depression will require treatment with antidepressant medication or psychological treatments as described in Chapters 2 and 3.

Review and offer referral from primary care

If symptoms have not responded to a logical escalation of treatment regimes (i.e. SSRI, dual action antidepressant such as venlafaxine, psychological treatment, combination treatment with medication and CBT) you should consider referral to a specialist mental health practitioner or service.

Summary

Mixed depression and anxiety is the most common form of mental illness you will see in primary care. Patients often present with somatic problems; we therefore argue that you should screen everyone you see with the depression and anxiety screening questions. Once diagnosis has been confirmed, treatment with SSRIs will be effective for most patients.

Melissa is 26 years old. She has been seeing the GP for a number of weeks now. He diagnosed severe mixed anxiety and depression and prescribed the SSRI fluoxetine. Melissa's symptoms did not improve at all so the GP tried another SSRI then switched to venlafaxine. The GP had referred Melissa to the IAPT worker but she did not go. Melissa has been brought in by her mother today. Her mother is concerned as Melissa is not eating or sleeping; a few days ago she said she was going to hang herself but has barely spoken since.

Melissa was verbally unresponsive to the GP's questions, nodding or shaking her head in response. On being asked if she would hang herself, she just shrugged.

The GP advised Melissa and her mother that she should be seen by the mental health team immediately; they agreed.

References

American Psychiatric Association (APA) (2000) *Diagnostic and Statistical Manual of Mental Disorders (DSM)*. 4th edn. Arlington VA: APA.

American Psychiatric Association (APA) (2010) *Proposed Diagnostic Criteria for Mixed Anxiety Depression*. Retrieved 1 August 2010 from American Psychiatric Association website: http://www.dsm5.org/ProposedRevisions/Pages/proposedrevision.aspx?rid=407 (last accessed: 24.4.11).

Singleton, N., Bumpstead, R., O'Brien, M. Lee, A. and Meltzer, H. (2001) *Psychiatric morbidity among adults living in private households,* 2000. Office for National Statistics.

Zigmond, A. and Snaith, R. (1983) The hospital anxiety and depression scale. *Acta Psychiatrica Scandinavica* **67**(6): 361–70.

Chapter 5

Depression and Anxiety in Long-term Conditions

In patients with long-term conditions such as diabetes, cardiovascular disease (CVD), stroke, or chronic obstructive pulmonary disease (COPD), depression and anxiety are very common co-occurring conditions. It is very easy to dismiss these symptoms as a normal reaction to a long-term illness: 'of course they are depressed they can't breathe.' We argue that effective treatment of co-morbid mental disorder in patients with long-term conditions can have a dramatic positive effect on clinical outcomes and must be taken more seriously by primary care practitioners.

Epidemiology

Depression is approximately two to three times more common in patients with long-term physical health problems than in people who have good physical health. In a recent study, 23 per cent of people with two or more chronic physical problems were rated as depressed versus 3.2 per cent of healthy controls (Moussavi *et al.*, 2007). Anxiety is also much more common in long-term conditions, for example in diabetes 49 per cent (Peyrot and Rubin, 1997), COPD 34 per cent (Yohannes *et al.*, 2006) and following a stroke 50 per cent (Wiart *et al.*, 2000). Whilst it might seem obvious that long-term conditions may be a cause or trigger for depression and anxiety, it is important to note that there is also evidence that mental health problems may in fact be a risk factor for physical illness, e.g. depression and cardiovascular disease, (Nemeroff, 2008).

Screening

The recognition of depression and/or anxiety in patients with a long-term physical condition is more complex than in those presenting with mental health problems alone. This is because some, particularly somatic, symptoms (such as fatigue, sleep disturbance, loss of appetite, poor concentration) can occur in both mental and physical disorders. So if a patient with a history of CVD presents complaining of 'fatigue', should you consider a mental cause or simply attribute the symptom to the longstanding physical problems that the patient is experiencing? In practice, healthcare professionals are biased towards a physical cause to explain symptoms and are often blinded to possible psychological reasons. Some authors have described this as diagnostic overshadowing.

We recommend that you follow the procedure for screening for anxiety and depression in all the patients you see with long-term conditions.

Step 1 – ask the two depression screening questions (described in Chapter 2).

Step 2 – ask the two anxiety screening questions (described in Chapter 3).

Step 3 – if the patient gives a positive (yes) response to both questions in step 1 and/or step 2 then you should ask three further questions to further improve the specificity of the assessment:

During the last month, have you often been bothered by:

- feelings of worthlessness?
- poor concentration?
- thoughts of death?

An additional measure that you may find helpful is the distress thermometer. This is a simple checklist assessment technique used in cancer care and other areas of physical health. It can be downloaded from:

http://www.epi.bris.ac.uk/ditit/pdf/3_DT%20Tool%20Revised.pdf
(last accessed: 2.1.12).

Treatment of depression and anxiety in long-term conditions

As you become more skilled at recognising and effectively treating co-occurring depression and/or anxiety in the patients you see with long-term conditions, then both their physical and mental wellbeing can be considerably enhanced.

There is evidence that antidepressants are safe and effective in the treatment of moderate to severe depression in long-term conditions, e.g. following a stroke (Wiart *et al.*, 2000), and in diabetes (Lustman *et al.* 2000). The evidence for the safety and effectiveness of psychological treatments in this population is less clear; it is perhaps assumed that CBT will be safe, and few researchers have therefore sought to establish this.

An important observation made by a number of authors is that patients with a co-morbid mental health problem are more likely to be more non-adherent to all prescribed medication compared to those who are mentally well. So alongside ensuring that their mental illness is treated, it is also important to ask about and emphasise the importance of adhering to all treatments that have been prescribed.

Summary

In this chapter we have considered how to identify depression and/or anxiety in your patients who are living with long-term conditions. Many mental health problems can be effectively managed in primary care and patients may benefit from receiving their care from a clinician who is known to them in a non-stigmatised environment.

Gladys is 73 years old. She has come to see the practice nurse for her annual diabetes health check. The practice nurse asked Gladys the depression screening questions to which Gladys replied positively. She asked Gladys if she would like help and Gladys said she would but wasn't sure if she could.

The practice nurse encouraged Gladys to talk and tell her what was troubling her the most. She was upset because her youngest son was moving away to a new job and that would mean she would have no close family in the town. The practice nurse asked Gladys how this would affect her. She admitted she wouldn't really miss her son as he rarely came round but knew he was there if there was an emergency.

Having identified her concern, the practice nurse was able to discuss with Gladys what kind of emergencies she was thinking about and make a plan of which agency or friend to contact. The practice nurse offered Gladys an appointment for two weeks time to see how she was feeling.

References

Moussavi, S., Chatterji, S., Verdes, E., Tandon, A., Patel, V. and Ustun, B. (2007) Depression, chronic diseases, and decrements in health: results from the World Health Surveys. *Lancet* **370** (9590): 851–58.

Lustman, P., Freedland, K., Griffith, L. and Clouse, R. (2000) Fluoxetine for depression in diabetes: a randomized double-blind placebo-controlled trial. *Diabetes Care* **23** (5): 618–23.

Nemeroff, C. (2008) Recent findings in the pathophysiology of depression. *Focus* **6**: 3–14.

Peyrot. M. and Rubin, R. (1997) Levels and risks of depression and anxiety symptomology among diabetic adults. *Diabetes Care* **20**: 585–90.

Wiart, L., Petit, H., Joseph, P., Mazaux, J.M. and Barat, M. (2000) Fluoxetine in early poststroke depression. A double-blind placebo-controlled study. *Stroke* **31**: 1829–32.

Yohannes, A.. Baldwin, R. and Connolly, M. (2006) *Age and ageing* **35** (5): 457–59.

Chapter 6

Dementia

Dementia is a term that is used to describe a number of discrete disorders that include Alzheimer's disease and vascular dementia. Perhaps the most prominent symptom of dementia is problems with short-term memory. Dementia patients may also have problems with thinking (cognition), language, understanding and judgement. Emotional lability and behavioural problems are also common, as are changes in personality. In the later stages of the illness, patients often become disoriented in time, place and person. Dementia is increasingly considered a long-term condition that can be effectively managed with medicine; it is however progressive and incurable.

Types of Dementia

Different dementias are characterised by different causes and symptoms. We shall briefly consider the most common forms of the illness.

Alzheimer's disease

Alzheimer's disease is the most common form of dementia affecting around half a million people in the UK (Alzheimer's Society, 2010). In Alzheimer's patients 'plaques' and 'tangles' develop in the structures of the brain leading to the death of brain cells. It has also been observed that there is a shortage of certain key neurotransmitters.

Alzheimer's is a progressive disease; over time, more of the brain is destroyed and symptoms become more severe. Common symptoms of Alzheimer's disease include:

- the early stages (typically the first few months):
  - lapses of memory and problems finding the right words;
- In the later stages (typically months to years):

- confusion: the patient frequently forgets people's names, places, appointments and recent events;
- mood swings: patients may be sad or angry, feel scared and frustrated by their memory problems;
- withdrawal and isolation, due either to a loss of confidence or to communication problems.

Vascular dementia

Vascular dementia is the second most common form of this illness, affecting around 200,000 people in the UK. Vascular dementia is caused by impaired blood flow to the brain, either from narrowing or complete blockage of blood vessels, depriving cells of nutrients and oxygen, eventually destroying them. Narrowing of blood vessels is caused by conditions such as diabetes and hypertension. Blockage is typically the result of several small strokes that occur repeatedly over time or follows a major stroke. Because of the different causes of vascular dementia, symptoms may develop suddenly and quickly worsen, or they may develop gradually over many months. Common symptoms of vascular dementia include:

- memory loss
- difficulties with tasks that require concentration and planning
- depression
- changes in personality and mood
- episodes of confusion
- urinary incontinence
- poor attention
- stroke-like symptoms, such as paralysis on one side of the body
- slow and unsteady gait
- night time wandering.

Dementia with Lewy bodies

Dementia with Lewy bodies is characterised by deposits of the protein alpha-synuclein inside brain cells. These deposits are called Lewy bodies, named after Friedrich H. Lewy, who described them in the early 1900s. Affecting around 30,000 of the UK population, disease progression is difficult to characterise. In some patients symptoms develop progressively at a steady rate; in others decline can be profound and dramatic. The common symptoms of dementia with Lewy bodies include:

- memory loss
- poor attention span
- episodes of confusion
- delusions
- difficulty in planning
- muscle stiffness
- slowed movement
- shaking and trembling of limbs
- shuffling gait
- sleep problems
- loss of facial expression
- visual hallucinations.

Frontotemporal dementia

Affecting around 15,000 people in the UK, frontotemporal dementia is a rare form of dementia usually occurring in patients between 50 and 60 years of age. It is caused by damage to the frontal or temporal lobe of the brain which controls emotional responses and behaviour. As a consequence many of the initial symptoms of frontotemporal dementia involve changes in emotion, personality and behaviour. Patients with this form of dementia may become less sensitive to other people's emotions, which can make them appear selfish and unfeeling. They may become disinhibited which can lead to 'inappropriate' behaviour, for example making sexually suggestive gestures in a public place, being rude to others or making tactless comments (e.g. 'you're fat, aren't you?', 'I don't like your jogging trousers!'). Other symptoms of frontotemporal dementia include:

- aggression
- compulsive behaviour
- being easily distracted
- lack of interest in personal hygiene
- change in personality.

Frontotemporal dementia can also cause problems with language and patients may have problems finding the right words to express themselves. So they may use many words instead of a few to describe something. For example a patient might say, 'a wooden utensil with handles used for making pastry' instead of 'a rolling pin'.

It is important to note that in this form of dementia, the patient's memory often remains intact.

Diagnosis and assessment

To make a dementia diagnosis you will need to undertake a comprehensive assessment. Typically this will include:

- A detailed medical history.
- Medication reconciliation to identify any drugs that may impair cognitive functioning.
- Full physical examination.
- Blood tests (full blood count, calcium, glucose, renal and liver function, thyroid function tests, serum vitamin B_{12} and folate levels). If delirium is a potential differential diagnosis then perform a midstream urine test to rule out infection. You should also consider a chest X-ray (to rule out chest infection causing delirium) and an electrocardiogram (ECG) as determined by the patient's clinical presentation.
- Clinical cognitive assessment. This should include examination of attention and concentration, praxis, orientation, language, short- and long-term memory, executive function. It is also important to take into account other factors that may affect cognition such as educational attainment, prior level of intellectual functioning, language abilities and sensory impairment.
- Standardised measures of cognitive functioning:
  - The 6-Item Cognitive Impairment Test (6-CIT) (Brooke and Bullock, 1999). The Kingshill Research Centre owns the copyright to the Kingshill Version 2000 of the 6-CIT but allows free usage to healthcare professionals. You can access and complete it on line at: **http://www.patient.co.uk/showdoc/40026041/** (last accessed: 2.1.12).
  - Mini Mental State Examination (MMSE) (Folstein *et al.* 1975). This has to be purchased from the current copyright holders, Psychological Assessment Resources.
  - General Practitioner Assessment of Cognition (GPCOG) (Brodaty *et al.*, 2002).

- The 7-Minute Screen (Solomon 2000).
- Assessment of psychiatric co-morbidities, including depression and psychosis.

It is important to ask patients who are being assessed for possible dementia whether they wish to know the diagnosis and with whom (if anyone) it should be shared.

Memory assessment services

Patients with suspected dementia should be referred to your local memory assessment service. This service will provide:

- a comprehensive assessment
- confirmation of diagnosis
- initiation of treatment
- provision of information, advice and support to families and carers
- signposting of patients and carers to social care and voluntary organisations that provide additional support and services.

Treatment

There is good evidence that a combination of drug and psychological treatments can be effective in dementia. They include:

- Acetylcholinesterase inhibitors (we provide a detailed description of these medicines in Chapter 10).
- For people with mild-to-moderate dementia, a structured group cognitive stimulation programme can be beneficial.
- Non-medical interventions tailored to the person's preferences, skills and abilities, such as aromatherapy, music and/or dancing, pet therapy or massage may be valued by patients.

Annual review

It is the patient's GP's responsibility to ensure that an annual face-to-face review is carried out (NHS Employers and BMA, 2011). The review should focus both on the health and social needs of the patient and their carer(s). Specifically the review should focus on the following:

- Physical and mental health:
  - Blood tests (full blood count, calcium, glucose, renal and liver function, thyroid function tests, serum vitamin B_{12} and folate levels).

People with dementia often do not complain of common physical symptoms, but experience them to the same degree as the general population, and people with vascular dementia have the same CVD risk as those with stroke and diabetes. By making these investigations you may pick up a cardiovascularcondition that you can treat and offer the appropriate CVD preventative intervention.

- Checking for concurrent physical conditions (e.g. joint pain or intercurrent infections).
- Review of new or emergent dementia symptoms (e.g. wandering).
- Screening for depression.

• If appropriate, provide the patient and the carer with information appropriate to the stage of the illness and the patient's health and social care needs.

• If the patient has a carer, discuss the impact of looking after the patient.

• If applicable you should communicate with and co-ordinate arrangements with secondary care.

• Where a number of agencies are involved, you should additionally focus on assessing the communication between health and social care and non-statutory sectors as appropriate, to ensure that potentially complex needs are addressed.

Summary

In this chapter we have considered the different forms of dementia that patients may present with. We have also reviewed the range of symptoms, beyond memory problems, that dementia patients can experience. Early diagnosis is essential to ensure that patients are able to access evidence-based treatment. The annual review is the responsibility of primary care practitioners and is key to ensuring that patients and carers are getting the information, support, care and treatment required for the effective management of this long-term illness.

Derek is 67 years old. When seeing the practice nurse for a blood pressure check he mentioned he was having some memory problems. The practice nurse asked him if he was worried about it. He replied that he was concerned that he was going senile. The practice nurse explained that she could carry out a simple test which may indicate whether he might have dementia and asked if he would like to take it. Derek said he would, so the practice nurse carried out the 6-CIT test. Derek scored 18/28 which meant that he had significant memory loss.

Derek was unsurprised by the result and asked what would happen next. The practice nurse gave details of the tests they would do in the health centre (ECG and blood tests) and then she would ask the GP to refer him to see a specialist.

References

Alzheimer's Society (2010) *What is Alzheimer's disease?* Online: http://www.alzheimers.org.uk/factsheet/401 (last accessed: 24.4.11).

Brodaty, H., Pond, D., Kemp, N., Luscombe, G., Harding, L., Berman, K. and Huppert, F.A. (2002) The GPCOG: a new screening test for dementia designed for general practice. *Journal of the American Geriatrics Society* **50** (3): 530–4.

Brooke, P. and Bullock, R. (1999) Validation of a 6 item cognitive impairment test with a view to primary care usage. *International Journal of Geriatric Psychiatry* **14** (11): 936–40.

Folstein, M., Folstein, S. and McHugh, P. (1975) 'Mini-mental state'. A practical method for grading the cognitive state of patients for the clinician. *Journal of Psychiatric Research* **12** (3): 189–98.

NHS Employers and British Medical Association (2011) *Quality and Outcomes Framework guidance for GMS contract 2011/12.* **http://www.nhsemployers.org/SiteCollectionDocuments/QOFguidanceGMScontract_2011_12_FL%20 13042011.pdf** (last accessed: 2.1.12).

Solomon, P. (2000) Recognizing the Alzheimer's disease patient: the 7 minute screen. *Revista Neurologica Argentina* **25** (3): 113–20.

Chapter 7

Sleep Disturbance

Most adults need to sleep for between seven and eight hours a night to feel refreshed. The quality of sleep is as important as the number of hours a person sleeps, if not more important. Inadequate or disturbed sleep can affect both a patient's physical and mental wellbeing. Are sleep problems mental, neurological or physical disorders? In many ways this is a superfluous question, certainly for those of us working in primary care where we have to treat whatever problems are presented to us by the patients that walk through the door. We decided to include a chapter on sleep disturbance in a book about mental health problems, not because sleep disorders are included in the *Diagnostic and Statistical Manual of Mental Disorders* (4th edition) but for pragmatic reasons; these are common and challenging problems that primary care practitioners are required to deal with on a daily basis.

What is sleep?

Sleep is essential to maintain cognitive skills such as speech, memory and thinking. There is a predictable pattern of sleep through the night (or day for night workers) that most people will follow. There are two main forms of sleep: REM (rapid eye movement, deep sleep) and non-REM (broken down into four different stages). How well rested the patient feels depends on how much of the various forms of sleep they get each night. Throughout sleep the brain stays active; each stage is linked to a distinctive pattern of electrical activity. Sleep usually begins by progressing over the course of an hour and a half, through the four stages of non-REM sleep; people then switch to REM sleep. After another 10 minutes they switch back from REM to non-REM sleep, repeating this cycle throughout the night with the REM sleep becoming longer each time. Table 7.1 describes REM and the four stages of non-REM sleep. It is important to note that as people age they need less deep sleep, so those aged over 60 typically may wake more easily after 3–4 hours.

Table 7.1 *The forms of sleep*

Form: Non-REM Sleep (90 minutes)	
Stage 1:	Light sleep; easily awakened; muscle activity; eye movements slow down.
Stage 2:	Eye movements stop; slower brain waves, with occasional bursts of rapid brain waves.
Stage 3:	Considered deep sleep; difficult to awaken; brain waves slow down more, but still have occasional rapid waves.
Stage 4:	Considered deep sleep; difficult to awaken; extremely slow brain waves.
Stage 4 is followed by Stage 3 then Stage 2	
Form: REM Sleep (10–60 minutes)	
Usually first occurs about 90 minutes after the person falls asleep; cycles along with the non-REM stages throughout the night.	
Eyes move rapidly, with eyelids closed.	
Breathing is more rapid, irregular, and shallow. Heart rate and blood pressure increase. Dreaming occurs. Arm and leg muscles are temporarily paralysed.	

Common sleep problems

The most common sleep problems (insomnia) that patients in primary care present with include: difficulty in falling asleep, frequent awakening throughout the night, early morning awakening and restless sleep that leaves them feeling unrefreshed. Hyposomnia is generally used to refer to a patient who does not get enough sleep; conversely hypersomnia refers to a patient who sleeps excessively. Often patients will talk about how their sleep problems make them irritable and agitated, impacting on work and social functioning. Poor concentration, making it hard to carry out routine or required tasks, is also a common complaint reported by patients with sleep problems. Other consequences of disturbed sleep include:

- unintentionally falling asleep during the day
- feeling tired all the time
- memory problems
- difficulty in making decisions
- clumsiness.

Older people often present in primary care concerned that they are sleeping less, unaware that fewer hours of deep sleep are required as you age.

Causes of sleep disturbance

Sleep problems can be caused by specific sleep disorders as well as by a range of physical, psychological, lifestyle, pharmacological and environmental factors.

Sleep disorders

The two most common sleep disorders are sleep apnoea and narcolepsy. Both require specialist treatment in secondary care; for primary care practitioners, the key task is one of recognition and knowing who to refer to.

Sleep apnoea is characterised by temporary stopping of breathing during sleep. Typically patients with this disorder will present complaining of snoring loudly and daytime sleepiness. Diagnosis can really only be confirmed by specialists in a sleep laboratory.

Falling asleep suddenly without warning is the characteristic symptom of narcolepsy. Patients with narcolepsy often have lived with the condition for many years before seeking help. Patients who have a diagnosis of narcolepsy confirmed will frequently present to primary care complaining of an irresistible urge to sleep. The majority of patients with narcolepsy will experience cataplexy (loss of muscle tone) and around half will experience hallucinations (at the onset of sleep or on awakening). Diagnosis needs to be made by a specialist.

In patients who present complaining of sleep disturbance it is important to rule out sleep disorders before you start treating the patient yourself. We suggest the following questions:

- **'Have you ever been told that your snoring is very loud?'**

If they answer positively, then consider sleep apnoea and refer to the sleep clinic.

- **'Have you ever experienced sudden episodes of overwhelming sleepiness during the day in which you could not stay awake?'**

If they have, then consider narcolepsy and refer to the sleep clinic.

Physical causes

Physical factors that are commonly associated with sleep disturbance include:

- acute infection
- acute and chronic pain
- being overweight or obese

- heart failure
- respiratory disease
- restless leg syndrome.

In patients with common acute infection such as influenza the amount of time spent sleeping will increase dramatically. It is not uncommon for people to express concern about this (particularly after they have taken over the counter 'flu treatments') as they have to be able to 'carry on'. An increase in the amount of sleep during acute illness is a normal and healthy part of the recovery process caused by the immune system's production of large quantities of particular types of cellular hormones called cytokines. Explaining that sleep is critical in helping them recover is important advice to give, although it is often advice that is not heard.

As with infection, acute and chronic pain can cause an increased need for sleep; advice that this is healthy and something that patients should not be concerned about is appropriate. Acute and chronic pain, being overweight or obese, heart failure and respiratory diseases can all be physical causes of sleeping too little (hyposomnia), a problem that generally does require intervention.

Mental and psychological causes

Stress, worry, anxiety and depression are mental and psychological problems that interfere with sleep generally causing hyposomnia.

Lifestyle and environmental causes

An extensive range of lifestyle factors can influence sleep, causing both hypo- and hypersomnia. These include:

- room temperature (too hot or too cold)
- excessive use of alcohol, nicotine or caffeine
- sleeping during the day
- irregular sleep programme (i.e. going to bed and getting up at different times during the day)
- before bed:
  - eating excessively
  - working
  - playing computer games
  - physical activity.

Environmental factors affecting sleep:

- noise
- lack of privacy
- smelly or damp room
- uncomfortable bed.

Medication

Many medicines can cause sleep disturbance as a direct side effect. Patients may complain of difficulty getting to sleep as well as sleeping too much or too little. Other medicine side effects may indirectly cause sleep disturbance, for example, medicines that cause itching, dry mouth, or gastrointestinal disturbance as a side effect.

Determining the cause of sleep disturbance

Having eliminated specific sleep disorders, careful identification of the cause(s) of sleep disturbance is required to guide appropriate intervention. As there are no checklists available to help you identify the specific factors causing the sleep disturbance, we suggest you ask specifically about each possible cause as we have listed above.

Four principles that promote good sleep:

1. Co-morbidity

Physical causes should be dealt with by treating the underlying condition, for example if pain is causing the problem, then carry out any necessary investigations and treat with appropriate analgesia. If the cause is emotional, for example, depression or anxiety, then these conditions need to be dealt with (see Chapters 2, 3 and 4).

2. Sleep hygiene

Helping the patient to discover the cause of their sleep disturbance may be all that is needed to sort out their problem. We have listed some tips to help patients:

- Minimise the noise while trying to sleep; *keep the windows and doors shut, buy ear plugs.*
- Sleep in the dark; *hang blackout curtains or blinds.*

- Ensure comfort while sleeping, *not too hot or cold, comfortable bed.*
- Reduce caffeine intake; *cut down on carbonated drinks, tea or coffee particularly in the evening.*
- Reduce the amount of alcohol that you drink, *particularly before bed.*
- Reduce smoking, *particularly before bed.*
- Avoid eating or drinking before sleep; *finish eating 2–3 hours before bed.*
- *Exercise regularly, but not before bed.*
- Relax before going to sleep; *for example, read or have a bath.*
- No daytime sleeping, *even if poor sleep the night before.*
- Get up at the same time each morning.
- Go to bed at the same time at night.
- Avoid lying in bed worrying about not sleeping; *get up and do something relaxing (read, listen to music).*

3. Medication review

If there is interrupted sleep or somnolence due to medication, then you may need to consider an alternative.

4. Medicine

Sometimes a short course of a hypnotic will be helpful.

5. **Some patients may benefit from a sleep diary to help them monitor their progress.** They can rate their sleep from 0 (poor quality sleep) to 10 (very good sleep). An example is illustrated in Table 7.2.

Table 7.2 *Sleep diary*

Day and date	Bedtime	Wake time	Quality of sleep (0–10)
Monday			
Tuesday			
Wednesday			
Thursday			
Friday			
Saturday			
Sunday			

You can give your patient a self-help guide to aid sleep, available to download from: **http://www.ntw.nhs.uk/pic/leaflet.php** (last accessed 2.1.12)

Persistent sleep disturbance

Patients with persistent sleep problems may benefit from CBT available through the IAPT service.

Summary

Sleep problems are common and impact on patients' physical and mental wellbeing. It is important to exclude specific disorders that require referral and specialist treatment during consultations with patients presenting with problems sleeping. Promoting good 'sleep hygiene' is often effective and should always be tried before reaching for medication. The use of hypnotic medicines can be helpful but really only affords a short-term solution and does not treat the underlying problems causing sleep disturbance.

Mick is 21 years old. He has been on holiday for ten weeks since finishing university and is due to start a new job in two weeks. He has come to the GP requesting sleeping tablets because he can't get to sleep at night. He is worried because he will need to get up at 7am to get to his new job on time.

The GP asks Mick about his sleep routine. Mick has been staying up until 3am and getting up around 11am over the holidays. During the last week he has tried to go to bed at 10pm but hasn't fallen asleep until the early hours. Because of this he has still got up at 11am. He says he has been even more tired so has had a nap in the afternoon.

The GP informed Mick how sleeping tablets were addictive and can have a hangover effect in the morning. He suggested that Mick went to bed at 11pm and set his alarm for 7am. Even if he has not slept he advised Mick that he must get up and must not nap in the day. He explained that eventually his body would adapt to the new rhythm.

Chapter 8

Severe Mental Illness

Severe mental illness (SMI) generally refers to conditions where psychosis (e.g. delusions, hearing voices) is present. All patients with a diagnosis of schizophrenia, bipolar disorder or other psychosis should be included on your SMI register. Up to 50 per cent of people who have an SMI are seen exclusively in primary care (NHS Employers and BMA, 2011). Consequently responsibility for monitoring mental health, physical wellbeing and ensuring that their social care needs are met lies with the primary care team.

Schizophrenia

Schizophrenia is a psychotic disorder characterised by positive, negative and cognitive symptoms. Positive symptoms include hallucinations (hearing voices or seeing visions), delusions (beliefs held strongly by the patient but not shared by people around them) and thought disorder (for example conversation jumping from one thought to a completely unrelated thought). Social isolation and withdrawal are examples of negative symptoms. Cognitive symptoms are very common and include problems in concentration and task planning. Schizophrenia is a long-term condition and life expectancy is reduced by around 20 years compared to the general population. About two-thirds of the excess mortality can be attributed to CVD and a third to suicide. The symptoms of schizophrenia often result in major social or occupational disturbance. For example few patients with schizophrenia are in employment.

Epidemiology

Schizophrenia is not a common illness, affecting approximately one person in a hundred at some point in their lives. There are probably around 250,000 people living with schizophrenia in the UK. This means that the typical primary care practice will possibly have between 70 and 100 patients with schizophrenia on their SMI register. Onset tends to be when patients are in their teens to early twenties, and although schizophrenia is equally common in men and women, men tend to develop the illness when they are younger than women. This may be explained by certain female hormones having a protective effect against schizophrenia. It is worth noting that in women there is a spike in the onset of schizophrenia just after the menopause.

Cause

Fifty percent of the cause of schizophrenia can be attributed to genetics. In identical twins, if one has schizophrenia there is a 1 in 2 chance that the other twin will also have the illness. Whilst this is an interesting piece of knowledge the fact that we can't change our genes means that it is the other 50 per cent of the cause of schizophrenia that is more important, because we can potentially do something about it. The other half of the 'cause' of schizophrenia may include problems at the time of birth, life stress, and substance misuse (particularly cannabis use). In fact one of the most powerful arguments for prohibition of cannabis is to try and prevent schizophrenia in people with a genetic susceptibility to the illness.

Diagnosis

DSM-IV diagnostic criteria for schizophrenia

Two or more of the following symptoms during a one-month period (or one of these if the delusions are bizarre or hallucinations are commentary style):

- delusions
- hallucinations
- disorganised speech (e.g. incoherence or derailed thinking)
- grossly disorganised or catatonic behaviour
- negative symptoms (e.g. avolition (loss of ability to motivate, choose or resolve), lack of planning, emotional blunting or poverty of speech)
- social or occupational dysfunction – disturbance in one or more major areas, such as work, self-care or interpersonal relationships
- continuous signs of disturbance for at least six months
- schizoaffective disorder and mood disorder with psychosis have been ruled out
- substance misuse or a general medical condition have been excluded

- if autistic disorder or another pervasive developmental disorder is present, then schizophrenia can only be diagnosed if prominent delusions or hallucinations are present for at least one month.

Early detection of schizophrenia

Making a diagnosis of schizophrenia requires symptoms to be present for at least a month. Most GPs and psychiatrists are hesitant in giving patients a schizophrenia 'label' because of concerns about getting the diagnosis correct and because of the stigmatising effects of being placed on an SMI register. That said, early detection and treatment by the primary care team is essential in order to ensure that patients are effectively treated as quickly as possible. GPs or practice nurses are frequently the patient's first point of contact with a health professional. Intervening early can improve the outcome of the illness and can reduce the risk of suicide. Early schizophrenia often starts with increasing social isolation (not coming out of the bedroom) and deterioration in intellectual functioning. It is not uncommon for the families of people that go on to develop schizophrenia to talk about odd, strange, or unusual behaviour during their early years. It is often only when signs of psychosis emerge that patients come into contact with healthcare professionals.

Screening for schizophrenia

There are a number of tools that can be used to help screen for schizophrenia. One example is the PRIME early psychosis/schizophrenia screening test developed at Yale University in the USA (Miller *et al.*, 2003). (It can be downloaded from **http://www.schizophrenia.com/sztest/primetest.pdf** (last accessed: 2.1.12). This is a self-administered test; patients indicate to what extent they agree with 12 statements about their mental wellbeing. Statements include:

- I think that I have felt that there are odd or unusual things going on that I can't explain.
- I have thought that it might be possible that other people can read my mind, or that I can read others' minds.
- I think that I may hear my own thoughts being said out loud.

If you don't use a specific schizophrenia screening tool, it is important if you suspect a patient may be experiencing psychotic symptoms, to ask the following questions:

- Do you think that people are talking about you, watching you or criticising you?
- Can you see or hear things that other people can't?
- Do you feel that you have special powers?
- Do you think that you are particularly important?

Alternative explanations for psychotic symptoms

It is essential to consider non-psychiatric causes of psychosis. These include:

- systemic infections
- liver function disorders
- drug/substance intoxication
- drug withdrawal
- metabolic disorders
- nutritional deficiencies
- central nervous system abnormalities.

In short, our advice is that a physical health review is required in patients experiencing psychotic symptoms to exclude a possible physical cause.

Early Intervention Teams

Most secondary care mental health providers offer some form of early intervention service for patients with suspected psychosis. If you think a patient has psychosis you should refer them to this team of specialists as soon as possible.

Treatment

Schizophrenia is a long-term condition that requires treatment with antipsychotic medication to stabilise psychosis and prevent relapse of symptoms. Although many patients express a desire to come off medication, good adherence is essential to ensure effective management of the illness and psychosocial recovery. Antipsychotics are generally divided into two groups, typical and atypical. Typical antipsychotics are effective against psychosis for about eight out of ten patients but are associated with distressing movement side effects (restlessness, stiffness, dystonia) some of which can be irreversible (tardive dyskinesia). Newer atypical antipsychotics are as effective as the typicals but are associated with fewer movement side effects. Atypical antipsychotics have a different side effect profile that may include sedation, weight gain and sexual dysfunction. Some of the most frequently prescribed antipsychotics are considered in more detail in the medicines chapter.

Whilst antipsychotic medication is the foundation for the treatment of schizophrenia, talking treatments, particularly some forms of CBT and behavioural family therapy, may confer additional benefit in terms of symptom control.

Bipolar disorder

Bipolar disorder is a long-term condition characterised by episodes of elated mood (mania or hypomania) and depression. Symptoms are experienced by bipolar patients almost half of their lives and impaired personal and social function are common. Both diagnosis and effective treatment of bipolar are challenging. Substance use is extremely common and life expectancy is reduced in bipolar patients in part due to increased prevalence of CVD but also to very high rates of suicide.

Epidemiology

Estimates of the lifetime prevalence of bipolar disorder vary dramatically from study to study and range from around one to eight per cent. This variation can be attributed largely to problems in diagnosis. Peak age of onset is between 15 and 19 years of age.

Signs and symptoms of bipolar disorder

Mania

Mania is characterised by elated mood accompanied by increased drive, over activity and decreased need for sleep. There is increased speed of thought and this is expressed in pressure of speech. Initially, there may be enhanced productivity until efficiency is compromised by other symptoms such as poor concentration and distractibility. Irritability may occur rather than pure elation and can become a dominant symptom.

- Hallucinations and mood-congruent delusions occur in nine out of ten patients.
- Loss of social inhibitions and extravagant plans may result in grave consequences for an individual's professional life, social functioning and financial stability.
- Mania often results in such a severe disruption of functioning that hospital admission is necessary, sometimes requiring compulsory detention.

Depression

This manifests as low mood, loss of interest and enjoyment, diminished energy, poor concentration and disturbed sleep and appetite. Self-esteem and confidence are low. Ideas of guilt, hopelessness and suicide may occur. The diagnostic criteria are the same as those for unipolar major depression. Psychotic symptoms may feature in severe episodes and are typically mood congruent.

In comparison to unipolar depression, bipolar depression is more likely to present with psychomotor retardation, melancholic symptoms such as worthlessness, psychosis and atypical features such as hypersomnia. Bipolar depressive episodes are typically shorter than in unipolar depression. Patients presenting with depression directly following mania may be less likely to respond to treatment.

Mixed states

Some patients can experience a mixed emotional state, mania and depression, for example laughing hysterically and crying at the same time.

Diagnosis

In DSM-IV, bipolar disorder is divided into type I and type II.

Type I: episodes of mania with or without episodes of depression (though in reality depression commonly occurs).

Type II: episodes of hypomania (elevated mood but patients are able to function) and depression.

DSM-IV criteria for a manic episode

A distinct period of abnormally and persistently elevated, expansive or irritable mood, lasting one week (or any duration if hospitalisation is necessary). During the period of mood disturbance, three or more of the following symptoms have persisted (four if the mood is only irritable) and have been present to a significant degree:
- Increased self-esteem or grandiosity.
- Decreased need for sleep (e.g. feels rested after only three hours of sleep).
- More talkative than usual or pressure to keep talking.
- Flight of ideas (a rapid flow of thought, manifested by accelerated speech with abrupt changes from topic to topic) or subjective experience that thoughts are racing.

- Distractibility (attention too easily drawn to unimportant external stimuli).
- Increase in goal-directed activity (socially, at work or school, or sexually) or psychomotor agitation (relating to movement or muscular activity associated with mental processes).
- Excessive involvement in pleasurable activities that have a high potential for painful consequences (such as engaging in unrestrained buying sprees, sexual indiscretions or foolish business investments).
- The symptoms do not meet the criteria for a mixed episode.
- The mood disturbance is sufficiently severe to cause a marked impairment in occupational functioning or in usual social activities or relationships with others, or to necessitate hospitalisation to prevent harm to self or others, or there are psychotic features.
- The symptoms are not due to the direct psychological effects of a substance or a general medical condition.

DSM-IV criteria for depression are listed in Chapter 2.

Diagnostic challenges in bipolar disorder

Seven out of ten patients with bipolar disorder have been misdiagnosed at least once. Making a bipolar diagnosis is relatively easy when patients present in a manic state. However, most patients with bipolar disorder will present to primary care depressed (not manic) and it is all too easy to diagnose and treat the patient as if they had a unipolar depression. Treating patients with bipolar depression with antidepressant medication can be disastrous, potentially 'flipping' the patient into mania. We therefore strongly recommend that you ask every patient that you see who is presenting with a depressive disorder (and ideally available family members):

Have you ever experienced periods in your life where you have:
- been particularly talkative and/or irritable?
- been more active and/or productive than usual?
- felt elated and/or invincible?

If you suspect that a patient may have a bipolar rather than unipolar illness you can test this using the Mood Disorder Questionnaire (MDQ). The MDQ has 17 items and is completed by the patient. In trials the MDQ was shown to be accurate in detecting seven out of ten patients with bipolar disorder. You can download the MDQ from the following website: **http://www.dbsalliance.org/pdfs/MDQ.pdf** (last accessed: 2.1.12).

Early intervention

As in the treatment of schizophrenia early intervention in patients with bipolar disorder can be effective in improving long-term outcomes. Early intervention teams tend to be reluctant to make a firm bipolar diagnosis primarily because of concerns around stigma. This concern must however be balanced against the long-term nature of the condition and the need to ensure the patient is prescribed with and adheres to effective treatment.

Treatment

Bipolar disorder is a long-term mental illness that requires treatment with medication to:

- treat depression
- prevent depressive symptoms returning
- treat mania
- prevent manic symptoms from returning.

The most frequently prescribed medicines for bipolar disorder are lithium, carbamazapine and sodium valproate. Often these drugs are described (probably incorrectly) as 'mood stabilisers'. We would actively encourage you to disregard what you think you know about the treatment of bipolar disorder and consider what evidence has shown about the relative merits of different medicines.

Treatment of bipolar depression:

- Consider quetiapine or lamotrigine.

Prevention of depression symptoms returning (if depression is the predominant symptom):

- Consider quetiapine or lamotrigine.
- Consider lithium as a second line treatment.

Treatment of bipolar mania:

- Consider antipsychotics, valproate, lithium or carbamazapine (all are equally effective against mania; the choice would therefore be based on tolerability and the potential for drug interactions).

Prevention of manic symptoms returning (if mania is the predominant symptom):

- Consider lithium, aripiprazole, quetiapine, valproate or olanzapine.

- Consider carbamazapine as a second line treatment.

The pharmacological treatment of bipolar disorder is challenging, many patients requiring combination treatment with more than one medication. The most comprehensive summary of the state-of-the-art in terms of bipolar treatment is provided in the British Association of Psychopharmacology Guidelines **(http://www.bap.org.uk/pdfs/Bipolar_guidelines.pdf** (last accessed: 2.1.12)). In our experience the majority of patients are prescribed more than one medicine for their bipolar disorder. Often a treatment regime will evolve based on a process of trial and error. Bipolar disorder is certainly an aspect of mental health practice that requires research investment to inform practice.

Psychological therapies

As an addition to medication, psychosocial treatments – including certain types of talking therapy – are helpful in providing support, education, and guidance to people with bipolar disorder and their families. Psychosocial interventions can lead to increased mood stability, fewer hospitalisations, and improved functioning in several areas. Psychological therapies that have been found to be helpful include:

Cognitive behavioural therapy
CBT helps people with bipolar disorder learn to change inappropriate or negative thought patterns and behaviours associated with the illness.

Psycho-education
Psycho-education involves teaching people with bipolar disorder about the illness and its treatment, and how to recognise signs of relapse so that early intervention can be sought before a full-blown illness episode occurs. It may also be helpful for family members.

Family therapy
Family therapy uses strategies to reduce the level of distress within the family that may either contribute to or result from the patient's symptoms. It also aims to make the family an active part of the therapeutic structure.

Summary

Both schizophrenia and bipolar disorder are relatively uncommon but severe mental illnesses. Psychosis is a common feature of both disorders. Accurate diagnosis is essential to ensure that patients are getting appropriate and effective treatment. Long-term conditions such as schizophrenia and bipolar disorder require medication both to treat the acute symptoms and to prevent relapse. There is good evidence that some forms of psychological therapy can be useful adjuncts but not alternatives to drug treatment.

Adesh is 18 years old and has been brought into the surgery by his mother. She is concerned because over the last six months he has become increasingly withdrawn and is spending most of his time in his room. She says he used to have lots of friends but now he doesn't see anyone. He has stopped going to college which he used to enjoy.

The GP observes that Adesh is sitting quietly and has paid no attention to what his mother was saying. The GP asks Adesh how he is feeling; he does not look up and just shrugs. The GP asks him if he could hear or see anything that others could not. Adesh nods and says someone talked to him all the time. On seeing that Adesh is beginning to get distressed the GP decides not to question him any further but asks if he would like to see someone who may be able to help him manage the voice talking to him. Adesh nods.

The GP contacts the early intervention team by phone; they agree to see Adesh at home the next morning.

References

American Psychiatric Association (2000) *Diagnostic and Statistical Manual of Mental Disorders (DSM)*. 4th ed. Arlington VA: APA.

Miller, T., McGlashan, T., Rosen, J., Cadenhead, K., Ventura, J., McFarlane, W., Perkinds, D.O., Pearlson, G.D. and Woods, S.W. (2003). Prodromal assessment with the structured interview for prodromal syndromes and the scale of prodromal symptoms: predictive validity, interrater reliability, and training to reliability. *Schizophrenia Bulletin* **29** (4): 703–15.

NHS Employers and British Medical Association (2011) *Quality and Outcomes Framework guidance for GMS contract 2011/12*.

http://www.nhsemployers.org/SiteCollectionDocuments/QOFguidanceGMScontract_2011_12_FL%20 13042011.pdf (last accessed: 2.1.12)

Chapter 9

Monitoring the Physical Health of People with Severe Mental Illness

SMI is associated with high medical co-morbidity; life expectancy is reduced by up to 25 years compared to the general population. The major cause of death is cardiovascular disease. The 'average' patient with SMI in the UK has a BMI of around 30 (which is on the borderline of obese) compared with 25 in the general population (the borderline of overweight). The causes of obesity in these patients are multi-factorial and include unhealthy diets and lack of exercise. Some antipsychotic medications used to treat the psychiatric symptoms are also associated with weight gain. CVD risk factors that are also common in SMI patients include smoking, alcohol use, diabetes (which is more common in patients with schizophrenia), dyslipidemia and hypertension.

Other physical health problems are also common in patients with SMI. These include problems associated with:

- poor hygiene: fungal, urinary tract, skin, vaginal and genital infections, dental caries;
- sexual health: HIV, chlamydia, hepatitis B, gonorrhoea, genital warts;
- smoking: COPD, chest infections, pneumonia;
- cancer: self-examination, cervical, mammography, bowel screening.

Whilst patients with SMI attend primary care more frequently than the general population, their physical health problems seem to go unrecognised. This may be attributed to diagnostic overshadowing; symptoms that patients present with are automatically attributed to mental illness and clinicians fail to consider possible physical causes.

You should invite patients with SMI to have an annual physical health check to monitor CVD risk factors and offer appropriate health promotion and prevention advice (diet, exercise, smoking, self-examination, sex and substance and alcohol use). A physical health check also affords the opportunity to check patients' mental wellbeing, review their psychiatric medication and enquire about their social circumstances. We have produced a detailed guide for undertaking a physical health check – the HIP-PC – in patients with mental health problems that can be downloaded from the following website: **http://www.changingmindscentre. co.uk/resources//HIP-PC_2nd_ed[1]..pdf** (last accessed 3.1.12). The HIP-PC covers aspects of physical health that are particularly relevant in patients with mental health problems. The following is a précis of the HIP-PC.

Cardiovascular risk factors

Body Mass Index (BMI)

BMI is a proxy measure of body 'fatness' calculated using the formula weight divided by height squared. The following BMI categories are widely used and considered indicative for both men and women: below 18 suggests a person is underweight, 19–24 is optimum, 25–29 overweight and more than 30 obese. Although BMI is widely used, it can be misleading in people who are athletes or who weight-train or in pregnant or breastfeeding women and in those over the age of 60 years. BMI categories vary slightly according to ethnicity. This is particularly noteworthy in patients of South Asian origin where overweight is considered to be a BMI of 23 to 24, and obese above 25. As in the general population, overweight and obese patients with SMI require intervention to encourage weight loss. There is evidence that interventions, for example, using motivational interviewing techniques, can be effective in facilitating changes in diet and exercise that may lead to weight loss. It is worth noting that it may take more time and require more intensive input to enable these patients to lose weight.

Waist circumference

Waist circumference in the general, but perhaps more so in the SMI, population is an important measure of body fatness. People who carry their excess fat centrally (within the abdominal cavity) are more likely to develop CVD. In women a waist circumference above 80cm and in men above 94cm suggests patients are overweight and intervention is required.

Pulse rate

Tachycardia (a rapid heartbeat) is a symptom of a number of cardiovascular illnesses that include atrial fibrillation. It is also a common side effect of antipsychotic medications (particularly clozapine). An electrocardiogram (ECG) should be considered for all patients taking antipsychotics, but is a necessity for those prescribed high doses of antipsychotic medication or with an increased pulse above 100 beats per minute.

Blood pressure

The British Hypertension Society Guidelines cite evidence that suboptimal blood pressure control leaves patients at an unacceptably high risk of CVD complications and death, particularly from coronary heart disease (CHD) but also from stroke. You should check blood pressure, and then follow the British Hypertension Society guidelines.

QRISK®2

We also recommend that you check overall CVD risk using QRISK®2 (Hippisley-Cox et al., 2008).

Blood tests

Liver Function Tests (LFTs)

Because alcohol and substance use are highly prevalent and patients are generally on long-term antipsychotic medication it is important to check liver function. Early detection of hepatic disease can prevent further serious complications.

Lipid Levels

Dyslipidemia is an important risk factor for CVD and is prevalent in SMI patients. A fasting test is only required if cholesterol/HDL ratio is raised.

Glucose

Diabetes occurs in 15% of people with schizophrenia compared to only 5% of the general population. A fasting test is only required if the glucose level is raised to rule out or confirm impaired glucose tolerance or diabetes.

Prolactin

Hyperprolactinaemia is a common side-effect of many antipsychotic drugs. Symptoms include gynaecomastia, galactorrhoea, amenorrhoea and sexual dysfunction. Switching to a prolactin sparing antipsychotic has been shown to lead to normalisation of serum prolactin and resolution of the symptoms. You should monitor proactively for hyperprolactinaemia by checking patients' prolactin. In patients with raised prolactin levels the following is recommended (Peveler *et al.*, 2008):

- <1000 mIU/L (~50 ng/mL)) – continue to monitor.
- >1000 mIU/L (~50 ng/mL) – consider switching to an antipsychotic medication with a lower potential to elevate prolactin if this can be achieved safely.
- > 3000 mIU/L (~150 ng/mL) then a prolactinoma should be considered. If the levels do not return to normal upon switching to a less prolactin elevating antipsychotic, or if such switch is not possible for clinical reasons, then referral to a specialist in endocrinology is warranted to exclude a prolactinoma.

  An urgent referral is required if there are symptoms or signs of optic chiasmal compression (e.g. hemianopia, headache).

Urea and Electrolytes (U&Es) and calcium

For patients taking lithium, there is a higher than normal incidence of hypocalcaemia, and abnormal renal function. For patients taking lithium, six monthly checks are recommended.

Thyroid Function Test

For patients taking lithium, there is a higher than normal incidence of hypothyroidism. For patients taking lithium six monthly checks are recommended.

Full Blood Count (FBC)

Leukopenia and neutropenia are recognised as potential side effects of antipsychotic medication therefore we also recommend that you check FBC in the presence of symptoms (e.g. repeated infections).

B¹² and Folate

Having a deficiency of vitamin B^{12} because of a poor diet is rare in Western countries. Unhealthy diets are common in patients with schizophrenia. We therefore recommend that you check vitamin B^{12} and folate in all SMI patients.

Lithium

There are toxic effects of lithium (primarily used to treat bipolar disorder) at serum levels above 1.5 mmol/L. At levels above 2.0 mmol/L disorientation and seizures commonly occur that typically progress to coma and ultimately death. The therapeutic lithium level is between 0.4 and 0.75 mmol/L (this can vary from laboratory to laboratory). For patients stabilised on lithium therapy, levels must be monitored every three months.

Screening

Cervical cytology

Women with schizophrenia have a lower cervical cancer screening rate than the general population. If the patient has had no recent cervical cytology and has been sexually active, then you should offer her education and screening.

Testicles check

Testicular cancer is one of the most common cancers in men between the ages of 16 and 35 years. Self-checking is important; we might expect, but don't know for certain, that patients with SMI are worse than men in the general population at checking. Pragmatically it may be helpful to provide information on signs and symptoms of testicular cancer and actively encourage testicular self-examination.

Teeth

The dental health of patients with severe mental illness is notoriously poor. Compliance with a good oral hygiene routine tends to be lax and consumption of high sugar diets is common. Access to NHS dentists is also challenging and private treatment can be extremely costly. Antipsychotics, antidepressants and mood stabilisers can increase the risk of dental disease by causing a reduced saliva flow leading to caries, gingivitis and periodontal disease. Patients should be actively and repeatedly encouraged to visit a dentist.

Eyes

Antipsychotic medication may cause lens and cornea damage, and has been associated with cataract development. Patients with severe mental illness should be encouraged to routinely visit a local optician.

Feet

Some patients with severe mental illness struggle to maintain their personal care. Lack of proper care, ill-fitting shoes and general foot neglect are responsible for the majority of foot problems. You should exchange information on keeping feet healthy, e.g. washing daily, trimming nails, treatment for burns, cuts and breaks in the skin.

Breast examination (women and men)

Breast cancer is the most common cancer in the UK. Although there is no evidence of an increase risk of breast cancer in patients with SMI, hyperprolactinaemia can lead to breast-related problems. Ask about any symptoms (painless lump, nipple discharge, ulceration or swelling) and advise patients on self-examination.

Menstrual cycle

Hyperprolactinaemia can cause amenorrhoea. It is important to take a detailed history of the patient's menstrual cycle. If the patient has amenorrhoea, you should consider offering an oral contraceptive if this is not contraindicated, to reduce the risk of subsequent osteoporosis or switching antipsychotic medication to one that is prolactin sparing.

Lifestyle

Sleep

Sleep problems are extremely common in patients with untreated psychiatric symptoms. Psychotropic medication can affect the amount (for example sedation is a common side effect) and quality of sleep (increased dreaming is reported in patients taking some antipsychotic medications). You should clarify any sleep problems and provide education on good sleep hygiene.

Smoking

People with SMI have higher rates of smoking than the rest of the population; in fact around eight out of ten patients smoke. You should give advice about the possible health risks associated with smoking, ask about respiratory symptoms and perform a chest examination if appropriate. You can refer any patients wishing to quit smoking to NHS Stop Smoking Services, but it may be more appropriate to support them individually. You must review their medication first as cigarette smoking lowers the levels of some antipsychotic medications. Blood levels of olanzapine and clozapine should be measured before a patient stops smoking. A 25% dose reduction during the first week of cessation is generally recommended. Bupropion (Zyban) as a smoking cessation aid is contraindicated in bipolar disorder because of the risk of switch to mania.

Exercise

People with severe mental illness are considerably less active than the general population. A sedentary lifestyle is a risk factor for CVD. Exercise reduces CVD risk and also benefits patients' mental well-being. You should discuss their activity with the patient, and use positive encouragement to help them to increase their level.

Alcohol Intake

Consumption of more than 21 units of alcohol per week in women and 28 in men is a risk factor for CVD. Alcohol misuse is prevalent in patients with mental health problems. You should offer recommendations on sensible daily alcohol intake. If appropriate refer the patient to your local Alcohol Support Agency.

Diet

People with SMI often eat a poor diet, low in fruit and vegetables and high in fat. This contributes to poor physical and emotional health. You should aim to address the potential barriers, i.e. access and availability of fresh fruit and vegetables, awareness of health benefits and attitudes towards buying, preparing and eating fruit and vegetables. Then offer help with diet planning.

Fluid Intake

A balanced fluid intake is an important part of health. Patients with SMI commonly don't drink enough fluids. Overconsumption – polydipsia – is also a serious and common co-morbidity in patients with schizophrenia. You should determine patients' daily fluid intake and advise the patient to drink 1–2 litres (6–8 glasses) of fluid every day (more during hot weather and physical exertion).

Urine

Many medical conditions (urinary tract infection, diabetes, excess weight loss) can be detected by using medical urine test strips; therefore you should dip test urine annually using multistix diagnostic strips. Follow your usual protocols for abnormalities.

Bowels

People with schizophrenia are almost twice as likely to have bowel cancer as the general population and they seldom complain of gastrointestinal symptoms unless specifically asked. You should ask about symptoms and offer information on increasing physical activity, lowering alcohol and a healthy diet.

Caffeine intake

Caffeine can worsen psychotic symptoms. It is present in drinks such as coffee, tea and cola. If patients are drinking too many of these drinks, advise them to reduce caffeine intake, stopping gradually to avoid withdrawal effects.

Safe sex

Patients with SMI are more likely to engage in high risk sexual behaviours such as sex without a condom, anal sex and injecting drug use that may increase the risk of HIV infection. Other sexually transmitted infections that include chlamydia and gonorrhoea are also prevalent. You should provide sexual health advice as appropriate.

Sexual satisfaction

Antipsychotic medication can have an adverse effect on sexual function, which impacts greatly on quality of life. The main cause of sexual dysfunction in both men and women is hyperprolactinaemia. You should ask about this and carry out appropriate tests.

Cannabis

Cannabis use is associated with poorer outcomes in patients with schizophrenia and may precipitate psychosis in individuals with pre-existing liability. You should ask the patients about cannabis and other non-prescribed drug use during their physical health check.

Medication review

People with an established diagnosis of schizophrenia or bipolar disorder who are managed in primary care require monitoring of medication use, medication adherence and side effects. Side effects should be monitored in a systematic manner using a recognised tool such as the Side Effects Scale/Checklist for Antipsychotic Medication (SESCAM) which can be downloaded from **http://www. changingmindscentre.co.uk/v/tools** (last accessed: 24.4.11).

Vaccination

Flu vaccination

Patients with SMI are at an increased risk of cardiac, respiratory disorders and diabetes, therefore we recommend that you offer them annual immunisation against influenza.

Additional factors

Care plan

The Care Programme Approach (CPA) is the process which mental health service providers use to co-ordinate the care for people who have mental health problems. It is a condition of the General Medical Service contract to document a care plan in the patient's records; this care plan should be agreed between individuals, their family and/or carers as appropriate. If the patient with SMI does not receive any input from secondary care services, the primary healthcare professional should document an accurate and easily understood plan of care as part of the annual review by discussing this with the patient, family and/or carers.

Follow up

Patients may not attend for their health check when invited due to their mental state. It is therefore important to set up a robust system to increase the likelihood of attendance and allow further opportunities to attend. If the patient has a known carer or community mental health worker, you could inform them of the invitation at the same time. If the patient does not attend the annual review, you should follow this up with a telephone call to the patient, the patient's carer or community healthcare worker as appropriate, offering them another appointment. If this is not possible a further letter should be sent.

Summary

It is important to monitor the physical health of people with SMI to try to reduce their risk of CVD and to identify and treat any physical health problems that they would not report themselves. The annual health check also offers the opportunity to review the patient's medication, both benefits and side effects and to assess the patient's emotional wellbeing and social situation.

Adrian is 25 years old. He has come to see the practice nurse for his health check. He tells the nurse that he feels well. The practice nurse carries out a full examination and finds that he has athlete's foot. It is obvious to the nurse that Adrian hasn't washed his feet for some time. The practice nurse asks Adrian if his feet feel itchy or sore. He says they are really itchy and feel horrible.

The practice nurse says she can give him some cream to put on to help the itching but he would need to wash his feet with soap and water first and make sure they were nice and dry before applying the cream. Adrian says he can do this. The practice nurse gently suggests that when they are better if he is able to carry on with the washing then this might stop them getting itchy again.

The practice nurse also discovered that Adrian's diet was very poor. She decided to book another appointment to discuss it as she felt he had enough to remember with his feet instructions.

References

Hippisley-Cox, J., Coupland, C., Vinogradova, Y., Robson, J., Minhas, R., Sheikh, A. and Brindle, P. (2008) Predicting cardiovascular risk in England and Wales: prospective derivation and validation of QRISK2. *British Medical Journal* **336**: a332.

Peveler, R., Branford, D., Citrome, L., Fitzgerald, P., Harvey, P.W., Holt, R.I., Howard, L., Kohen, D., Jones, I., O'Keane, V., Pariente, C.M., Pendlebury, J., Smith, S.M. and Yeomans, D. (2008) Antipsychotics and hyperprolactinaemia: Clinical recommendations. *Journal of Psychopharmacology* **22** (2) Supplement: 98–103.

Chapter 10

Medicines

In this chapter we will discuss the commonly used medicines to treat depression, anxiety, schizophrenia, bipolar disorder, dementia and sleep disturbance.

Medicines used for depression

In patients with moderate to severe depression (i.e. those with a PHQ-9 score of 10 or more) antidepressant medications represent an effective treatment. In clinical trials about eight out of ten patients respond to treatment; most will report that their symptoms almost completely go away (i.e. they have gone into remission). Until fairly recently it was common practice to tell patients that it would take four to six weeks for an antidepressant drug to work. This is not true. Response to treatment with antidepressant medication generally occurs within one to two weeks. In mild depression (i.e. patients with a PHQ-9 score of less than 10) antidepressant medication does not work and should not be prescribed. In moderate to severe depression, patients will usually need medication to improve their concentration and lift their energy levels before they are able to engage in psychological treatments.

Selective Serotonin Reuptake Inhibitors (SSRIs)

Fluoxetine, citalopram, paroxetine and sertraline are the most frequently used medicines for the treatment of depression. Serotonin (along with noradrenaline and dopamine) is one of the principal neurotransmitters in mood disorders; it is hypothesised that depression is associated with a lack of serotonin. Antidepressant drugs exert their effect by boosting serotonin levels in the brain. SSRIs do this by inhibiting the reuptake of serotonin into the neurone effectively tricking the brain into producing more of the neurotransmitter.

The most frequent adverse effects associated with SSRIs are nausea, diarrhoea, dizziness, agitation, insomnia, tremor and sexual dysfunction. The risk of bleeding is increased in patients taking SSRIs. They should not, therefore, be prescribed to patients taking 'triptans', warfarin, heparin, non-steroidal anti-inflammatory drugs or aspirin.

A note about St. John's Wort: there is evidence from meta-analysis that St. John's Wort may be effective in the treatment of depression. However, evidence from more recent methodological trials casts doubt on this conclusion and would seem to indicate no additional benefit over placebo. In a recent three arm study by Rapaport *et al.* (2011), St. John's Wort was shown to be no more effective than placebo over depression, but carried a significant side effect burden comparable with the SSRI citalopram.

Second choice antidepressants

In the two in ten patients who fail to respond to SSRIs about half will respond to treatment either with a different SSRI or class of antidepressant. Alternative classes of antidepressants include:

- SNRIs (Serotonin and Noradrenalin Reuptake Inhibitors) such as venlafaxine and duloxetine
- Noradrenergic and Specific Serotonergic Antidepressants (NaSSA) – mirtazapine
- Tricyclic antidressants (TCA) such as amitriptyline and lofepramine (dosulepin is restricted to specialist use and should not be prescribed routinely in primary care because of an increased cardiac risk and toxicity in overdose).

Serotonin and Noradrenalin Reuptake Inhibitors

Venlafaxine inhibits the neuronal uptake of serotonin, norepinephrine, and dopamine in the central nervous system; it is structurally unrelated to other antidepressants. As venlafaxine has a different molecular structure it is a logical strategy to try with patients who have not responded to treatment with SSRIs. Venlafaxine has a relatively short half-life so should be administered in divided doses, two or three times a day. There is an extended release formulation of the drug that requires only once a day administration. Common side effects of venlafaxine include nausea, headache, sedation, dry mouth, dizziness, insomnia, constipation, nervousness, raised blood pressure, tiredness, sweating, reduced appetite and sexual dysfunction.

You should not prescribe venlafaxine if your patient has uncontrolled hypertension or a high risk of a serious cardiac ventricular arrhythmia. If they have established cardiac disease, then you can prescribe with caution. It is obviously important to monitor all patients' blood pressure regularly; if it remains increased then we advise either dose reduction or discontinuation.

Duloxetine is a dual action antidepressant. There is a risk of an increase in blood pressure, therefore this should be monitored. Some patients may experience unpleasant or distressing restlessness in which case you should stop the drug.

Noradrenergic and Specific Serotonergic Antidepressants (NaSSA)

Mirtazapine increases noradrenergic and serotonergic neurotransmission in the central nervous system. Its effectiveness is equal to that of SSRIs but usually has fewer sexual side effects. It has been argued that patients respond more rapidly to mirtazapine than the other antidepressants but this is probably due to the fact that sedation is a fairly common side effect. Some patients experience extreme drowsiness when first taking mirtazapine; if they do you should advise them not to drive or operate machinery. Do not be tempted to reduce the dose as the drowsiness is not related to the amount of mirtazapine taken and should wear off. Weight gain is a common side effect with mirtazapine and it is perhaps not a drug of choice in patients who are obese or suffer from bulimia. Ask your patients to look out for fever, sore throat, sore mouth or other signs of infection as these may be symptoms of a very rare side effect, reversible agranulocytosis. If they do experience any of these symptoms, you should stop their mirtazapine and take a full blood count.

Tricyclic antidressants

Whilst TCAs were breakthrough drugs when they were first introduced in the 1950s we can't really think of a good reason why you might preferentially choose to prescribe them now. TCAs are not well tolerated compared with more modern antidepressants. Common side effects, which tend to be dose related, include dry mouth, blurred vision, constipation, urinary retention, sedation and postural hypotension. In overdose TCAs are highly cardiotoxic. More generally TCAs can cause sinus tachycardia, paroxysmal hypertension, and ECG changes. If your patient has an established cardiovascular illness then it is advisable to monitor their blood pressure and perform an ECG. TCAs should probably be avoided in patients who have had a recent myocardial infarction or who have an arrhythmia (particularly heart block) as there appears to be an increased risk of mortality. We also suggest you avoid prescribing TCAs for patients with ischaemic heart disease as they can increase the risk of ventricular fibrillation.

If you prescribe your patient a sub-therapeutic dose TCAs (i.e. a dose below 100mg/day) and they show a clear clinical response you should be mindful that this is probably a placebo response and not associated with the drug.

Third line treatments

Agomelatine is a melatonergic agonist (MT1 and MT2 receptors) and 5-HT2C antagonist. Melatonin has a key role in synchronising circadian rhythms, which are known to be disturbed in depressed states. Agomelatine may therefore be useful when sleep is a problem. One of the key advantages of agomelatine is its low propensity to cause sexual dysfunction.

It is possible that some atypical antipsychotic medications, particularly aripiprazole, may be useful as an adjunctive treatment to antidepressants in patients who have failed to respond to antidepressant monotherapy.

Serotonin syndrome

Serotonin is something of a 'Goldilocks' neurotransmitter. If you have too little then you get depressed, too much and you are at risk of developing serotonin syndrome. Serotonin syndrome is potentially life threatening and requires immediate medical intervention. Symptoms can be divided into three clinical categories (mental state, neuromuscular features and autonomic instability), though not all patients will present with all the features. The first is a change in mental state and may include agitation, confusion, delirium, hallucinations, drowsiness and coma. Neuromuscular features are shivering, tremor, teeth grinding, involuntary twitching and overactive reflexes. Autonomic instability may include tachycardia, fever, hypertension or hypotension, flushing and diarrhoea and vomiting. In severe cases seizures, hyperthermia, rhabdomyolysis, renal failure and coagulopathies may occur. Theoretically any drug that works by elevating levels of serotonin can induce this syndrome. The greatest risk however, comes from patients taking, either accidentally or intentionally, a combination of drugs that increase serotonin. The starkest example of this is when a patient is taking an SSRI and an MAOI at the same time. The syndrome can also be induced when SSRIs are taken in combination with TCAs or St John's Wort.

Mild symptoms of serotonin syndrome (e.g. flushing, teeth grinding, tiredness, poor concentration, nausea) can be managed by stopping the SSRIs, offering supportive care, and treating with a benzodiazepine. Moderately and severely ill patients should be treated as an acute medical emergency.

The importance of sticking with treatment

In many patients depression is a long-term condition that requires maintenance treatment. Following a first depressive episode patients need to stick with antidepressants for at least six months after their mood has improved to minimise the risk of a relapse of their symptoms. Patients who have had two or more episodes of depression need to stick with treatment for at least two years after their depression has gone into remission. Continuous treatment over a number of years is probably necessary in patients who have had multiple episodes of depression.

Switching antidepressants

In some patients there will be a need to switch from one antidepressant medication to another. For example if a patient has been taking fluoxetine for six weeks and their mood has not improved you might make the decision to switch them to venlafaxine. You need to consider carefully how you do this because of the risk of serotonin syndrome. As a general rule you should gradually taper down the dose of the old antidepressant before starting the new drug. Abrupt withdrawal should always be avoided. You should check the prescribing guidelines for switching antidepressant medication. These can be accessed through: **http://www.cks.nhs. uk/depression/prescribing_information/prescribing_information/switching_ antidepressants#-403240** (last accessed: 3.1.12).

Stopping antidepressants

Missing doses or abruptly stopping antidepressant medication can induce a discontinuation syndrome (headache, dizziness, nausea, paraesthesia, anxiety, flu-like symptoms, and diarrhoea). It is advisable to ask the patient to reduce their dose of antidepressants gradually; the period of time taken to do this will vary depending on how long the patient has been taking them. For example, a course taken over eight weeks or longer should be reduced over four weeks, but patients wishing to stop long-term treatment may need to taper the dose down over a longer period. Reducing antidepressant medication usually involves halving tablets and alternate day administration. If you explain to your patients that dose-tapering is standard procedure in order to minimise the discontinuation symptoms and give them written instructions, they are more likely to take your advice. Alternatively, for your patients taking an SSRI or venlafaxine, you could switch to fluoxetine. Because fluoxetine has a long half life it has been associated with fewer discontinuation symptoms. Once the patient has successfully switched to taking fluoxetine, they can then stop it.

Promoting adherence

McIntyre *et al.* (2003) have suggested six strategies you can use in practice to enhance your patients' adherence to their treatment with antidepressants:

1. Provide general information on depression including common signs and symptoms.
2. Discuss the importance of taking medication as prescribed and the implications of missed doses.
3. Frequently enquire and educate patients about the type, severity and duration of side effects.
4. Tell patients to expect several weeks before symptoms improve; explore scepticism and resistance to therapy.
5. Anticipate patient misinformation and dysfunctional beliefs about the illness or the treatment process.
6. Instruct patients to continue taking medications when they are feeling better and describe the rationale for maintenance treatment.

Medicines used to aid sleep

Patients who are experiencing difficulty in sleeping (generally insomnia) will often ask for 'pills to help them'. In this section we will discuss the most appropriate use of medicines to treat sleep problems.

The first step in helping a patient with sleep problems is to assess possible causes and promote good sleep hygiene (see Chapter 7). Medication can be helpful in treating sleep disturbances but should be considered a treatment of last resort. Benzodiazepines, Z drugs, melatonin and antihistamines are effective treatments for sleep disturbance.

Benzodiazepines

With something of an undeserved reputation as drugs of misuse, benzodiazepines – diazepam, lorazepam, temazepam, nitrazepam – carefully prescribed can be very effective in treating sleep disturbance. Benzodiazepines exert their effect by potentiating GABA (gamma-aminobutyric acid), the same mechanism of action as alcohol. Benzodiazepines are helpful in treating insomnia in a number of different ways:

- helping the patient to get to sleep;
- prolonging the duration of sleep;
- preventing interrupted sleep.

The patient's sleep quality when taking benzodiazepines will tend to be poorer as they will have more light and less deep sleep. Patients can become tolerant to benzodiazepines within three to fourteen days of starting treatment. With continued treatment patients can easily develop a dependency on the drugs; consequently you should avoid prescribing more than a two week course. Temazepam tends to work more rapidly than nitrazepam and diazepam. Benzodiazepines should be avoided in patients with breathing problems or sleep apnoea syndrome. Common side effects of benzodiazepines include day time sleepiness and lightheadedness, confusion and ataxia, amnesia, aggression and muscle weakness. Less common side effects include headache, vertigo, hypotension, salivation changes, gastro-intestinal disturbances, visual disturbances, dysarthria, tremor, changes in libido, incontinence, urinary retention, blood disorders, jaundice, pain, thrombophlebitis and rarely apnoea.

Z Drugs

Use of benzodiazepines has largely been supplanted by so called Z drugs – zopiclone, zaleplon and zolpidem – that are as effective but do not seem to cause dependence. That said, they are not licensed for long-term use as dependence has still been reported in a small number of patients. In patients with marked neuromuscular respiratory weakness including unstable myasthenia gravis, respiratory failure or severe sleep apnoea syndrome, these medicines should be avoided. Perhaps the most common side effect reported by patients taking Z drugs is taste disturbance. Less common side effects include nausea, vomiting, dizziness, drowsiness, dry mouth and headache. In a very few patients amnesia, confusion, depression, hallucinations, nightmares, light headedness, co-ordination problems and sleep-walking have been reported.

Melatonin

A naturally occurring hormone, melatonin regulates circadian rhythms of the body. Licensed for the treatment of sleep disturbance, melatonin maybe particularly helpful in treating people over 55 years with persistent insomnia, helping the patient get back into a natural sleep pattern. Treatment should not be for more than three weeks and should not be prescribed to patients with an autoimmune disease. Common side effects include pharyngitis, back pain, headache and asthenia. Less commonly patients may experience abdominal pain, constipation, dry mouth, weight gain, drowsiness, dizziness, sleep disorders, restlessness, nervousness, irritability, sweating, flatulence, halitosis, hypersalivation, vomiting, hypertriglyceridaemia, aggression, agitation, fatigue, impaired memory, mood changes, hot flushes, priapism, increased libido, leucopenia, thrombocytopenia, muscle cramp, skin reaction, lacrimation, and visual disturbances.

Antihistamines

Patients who have mild sleep disturbance may find particular antihistamine medicines (specifically promethazine) are helpful, utilising the drugs' sedating side effects. An additional benefit may be that, although not as potent as benzodiazepines or Z drugs, antihistamines do not have the 'hangover' and morning drowsiness associated with these more widely used hypnotics. Long-term use should be avoided because of a risk of rebound insomnia when the medication is stopped. Promethazine should be avoided in patients with severe coronary artery disease. Common side effects of promethazine include headache, psychomotor impairment, and antimuscarinic effects such as urinary retention, dry mouth, blurred vision, and gastrointestinal disturbances.

Medicines used for people with dementia

Patients with dementia are often prescribed a number of different psychotropic medications that may include acetylcholinesterase inhibitors, benzodiazepines, antidepressants and antipsychotics. Ensuring adherence to treatment is important and particularly challenging in patients with dementia and attention should be given to ensuring that patients are on the simplest treatment regime possible.

Acetylcholinesterase inhibiting drugs

Acetylcholinesterase inhibiting drugs are used in the treatment of mild to moderate dementia, exerting their effect by increasing levels of acetylcholine, a key neurotransmitter involved in memory and thinking. Currently these drugs must be initiated by a secondary care dementia specialist. Slower rates of cognitive decline in up to half of patients taking acetylcholinesterase inhibiting drugs have been reported. The Mini Mental State Examination (MMSE; described in Chapter 6) should be used before the start of and at regular intervals during treatment to monitor effects; note again that medication is working if scores decrease more slowly rather than increase. Because of dose-related cholinergic side effects, treatment should be initiated at a low dose then titrated according to clinical response and tolerability. Acetylcholinesterase inhibiting drugs should be discontinued in those patients who appear not to be responding. A repeat of the cognitive assessment four to six weeks after discontinuation is recommended to assess deterioration; if decline occurs during this period, consideration should be given to restarting therapy.

There are currently three acetylcholinesterase inhibiting medicines licensed in the UK for the treatment of mild to moderate Alzheimer's disease:

- Donepezil (Aricept) may be particularly useful in treating patients with Lewy body dementia, severe Alzheimer's disease and vascular dementia. Initially the dose is 5mg once daily at bedtime, increased if necessary to maximum of 10mg daily. Side effects include nausea, dizziness, vomiting, hallucinations, agitation, muscle cramps and urinary incontinence.

- Galantamine (Reminyl) seems to be particularly useful in people with mixed dementia (Alzheimer's disease and vascular dementia). Initially the dose recommended is 4mg twice daily for four weeks increased to 8mg twice daily for four weeks; the maintenance dose is 8–12 mg twice daily. Side effects include nausea, vomiting, abdominal pain, weight loss, hallucinations, depression and muscle spasm.

- Rivastigmine (Exelon) also seems most effective against patients with Lewy body dementia. The starting dose is 1.5mg twice daily, increased in steps of 1.5mg twice daily at intervals of at least two weeks according to response and tolerance; usual range 3–6mg twice daily; maximum dose is 6mg twice daily; if treatment is interrupted for more than several days it should be retitrated from 1.5mg twice daily. Side effects include nausea, vomiting, increased salivation, extrapyramidal symptoms, agitation and anxiety.

Memantine

Licensed for patients with moderate to severe Alzheimer's, it is thought that memantine exerts its effect by blocking glutamatergic (NMDA) receptors and as such represents a novel approach to the treatment of the disease. Benefit in the treatment of mild to moderate dementia remains uncertain. The initial starting dose is 5mg a day, increased in incremental steps of 5mg at weekly intervals. The maximum dose is 20mg a day. Generally well tolerated, common side effects include constipation, hypertension, headache, hypertension, dizziness and drowsiness.

Behavioural and psychological symptoms in dementia (BPSD)

Antipsychotic drugs

Commonly prescribed to treat behavioural disturbance in patients with dementia, antipsychotics have been shown to increase the risk of stroke (Gill *et al.*, 2005, Hermann *et al.*, 2004) and a meta-analysis of randomised trials in patients with dementia showed that atypical antipsychotic drugs may be associated with a small increased risk of death compared with placebo (Schneider *et al.*, 2005). It has therefore been compellingly argued that the risks of these medicines outweigh the benefits.

Common reasons for antipsychotic use in patients with dementia include restlessness, irritability and aggression, emotional instability, and loss of inhibitions. Risperidone is the only antipsychotic licensed for short-term (maximum six weeks) management of persistent aggression in elderly people with Alzheimer's dementia. It is recommended that psychosocial interventions such as reminiscence should be used as an alternative to antipsychotic medication.

Benzodiazepines

As a very short-term (no more than two weeks) treatment for BPSD, benzodiazepines such as lorazepam or diazepam may be helpful. Long-term treatment should be avoided.

Medicines used to treat co-occurring conditions

Depression

Depression co-occurs in about a third of patients with dementia. Evidence supporting the use of antidepressants is rather weak. SSRIs would probably be the first line treatment choice. Fluoxetine may be helpful in patients with emotional lability which is common in patients with vascular dementia. Evidence for the use of CBT to treat dementia-related depression is also weak. IAPT services are unlikely to accept referrals of patients with depression co-morbid with dementia.

Anxiety

About 20 per cent of patients with dementia experience anxiety in response to their dementia symptoms. Effective in the short term, the continued use of benzodiazepines (side effects are summarised earlier in this chapter) may be helpful; long-term treatment should be avoided as efficacy appears to drop off dramatically.

Sleep problems in dementia

Hypnotics, benzodiazepines and Z drugs may be used for short periods to treat sleep problems that frequently occur in dementia patients. For example sleep reversal, where the patient is awake at night and sleeps during the day, is very common. Sleep could be a symptom of depression and it is important to carefully assess for depression symptoms (you should consider using the measures we have described in Chapter 2).

Medicines used to treat schizophrenia

A severe mental illness, schizophrenia requires treatment with antipsychotic medication to address psychotic symptoms and prevent relapse. The positive symptoms of schizophrenia, such as hallucinations and delusions, are believed to be caused by an excess of the neurotransmitter dopamine in the limbic region of the brain. Antipsychotics exert their effect by blocking the dopamine receptors in the brain. Negative symptoms, that include lack of motivation and social isolation, and cognitive symptoms (impaired attention and memory, difficulty in forward planning and problem solving) are associated with low levels of dopamine in the cortex.

Older, so called typical drugs such as haloperidol have diffuse effects blocking dopamine receptors throughout the brain. As a consequence these drugs often cause a range of dopamine-related side effects that include extrapyramidal symptoms (EPS). Newer atypical medicines are more selective for dopamine receptors in the limbic region of the brain and rarely cause EPS.

Typical antipsychotics including chlorpromazine, haloperidol, pimozide, prochlorperazine, sulpiride, flupentixol, fluphenazine, trifluoperazine and zuclopenthixol were first introduced in the 1950s. Although still commonly used, most patients with schizophrenia are now treated with atypical antipsychotic drugs that started to be introduced in the early 1990s. Atypical antipsychotics include olanzapine, quetiapine, risperidone and aripiprazole.

All antipsychotics (both typical and atypical) are, clinically, equally effective against the positive symptoms of schizophrenia. As might be predicted by their pharmacology, atypical medicines seem to be more effective in treating some of the negative and cognitive symptoms and may be more helpful in treating mood symptoms of schizophrenia.

About two in ten patients will fail to respond to treatment with antipsychotic medication (typical or atypical) and are deemed to have treatment resistant schizophrenia. These patients should be treated with a drug called clozapine. Effective in about half of all patients with refractory schizophrenia symptoms, clozapine is complex to use. In about one per cent of patients it can cause agranulocytosis; consequently patients will require regular blood monitoring and have to be registered with a clozapine patient monitoring service.

Side effects

Antipsychotic medicines can cause a number of side effects. Some are relatively easy to manage, other more complex.

Extrapyramidal Symptoms (EPS)

Defining antipsychotic drugs, EPS are common in patients prescribed typical drugs but relatively rare in those treated with atypicals (at standard doses). The best way to treat (or avoid EPS) is to prescribe patients an atypical antipsychotic.

- Dystonia is characterised by prolonged muscle contraction, resulting in twisting body motions, tremor and abnormal posture. Typically this occurs within 48 hours of starting treatment or increasing the dose of medication. It can be effectively treated with antimuscarinic medication (e.g. procyclidine).
- Akathisia (literally can't sit still) tends to occurs within hours to days of treatment being initiated. A particularly distressing side effect, akathisia requires urgent treatment as it is associated with an increased risk of suicide. Akathisia can be effectively treated with benzodiazepines or propanolol (but not procyclidine which doesn't work).
- Mimicking the symptoms of Parkinson's disease, stiffness and tremor

generally emerge within days to weeks of initiating treatment with anti-psychotic medication. The symptoms can be treated with an antimuscarinic drug (e.g. procyclidine).

- Tardive dyskinesia (TD) is a late onset (tardive) abnormal (dys) movement (kinesia) disorder. When treated with typical antipsychotics there is a five per cent per year chance of developing TD. In practice this means that the longer the exposure to typical medicines the more likely it is a patient will develop it. TD is often but not always observed in the patient's face. For example the patient's tongue may twist or contort or dart in and out of their mouth. Oddly many patients are unaware of dyskinesic movements and many mental health professionals are remarkably poor at detecting them despite the fact that the movements are so distinctive. Stopping medication is not an effective treatment and prescribing antimuscarinic medication can actually make TD worse. This fact is perhaps justification enough for prescribing atypical over typical antipsychotics to treat schizophrenia. Tetrabenazine and clozapine are probably the most effective treatments for TD.

Other common side-effects of antipsychotics include drowsiness, apathy, agitation, excitement, insomnia, convulsions, dizziness, headache, confusion, gastrointestinal disturbances, nasal congestion, dry mouth, constipation, difficulty with micturition and blurred vision. Less common side effects include precipitation of angle-closure glaucoma, cardiovascular symptoms, ECG changes, venous thromboembolism, menstrual disturbances, galactorrhoea, gynaecomastia, impotence, weight gain, blood dyscrasias, photosensitisation, contact sensitisation, rashes, jaundice, corneal and lens opacities and purplish pigmentation of the skin, cornea, conjunctiva, and retina.

The atypical antipsychotics are generally considered to be much better tolerated than other antipsychotic drugs. The most problematic side effects of risperidone are related to elevated levels of prolactin (sexual dysfunction, amenorrhoea, galactorrhoea). Others to look out for include weight gain, dizziness, postural hypotension. Patients may develop hyperglycaemia or sometimes diabetes, particularly with clozapine, olanzapine, and possibly quetiapine, therefore monitoring weight and plasma-glucose concentration is advised.

Neuroleptic Malignant Syndrome (NMS) is a rare and potentially very serious life threatening allergic reaction to antipsychotic medication. It generally presents with muscle rigidity, fever, autonomic instability and cognitive changes such as delirium.

Long-acting antipsychotic injections

Antipsychotics can be administered either orally (as a tablet, or with some drugs as a liquid or an orodispersible) or as an injection (either a short- or long-acting injection that works for several weeks). There are a number of reasons why injections may be prescribed instead of tablets:

- It is easier for some patients to have one injection fortnightly or monthly than remembering to take tablets every day.
- The exact amount of medication that the patient is prescribed will be taken.
- When a patient has malabsorption, an injection may be more effective.
- There is a steady therapeutic medication level from regular injections.
- There is protection from relapse beyond the time of the last injection.

Some patients may be discharged from secondary care and will need to attend primary care for their injection. These are our recommendations for the practice nurse in terms of the effective administration of long-acting antipsychotic medicines:

- Follow the instructions provided with each particular injection.
- Give the dose as prescribed in the patient's records. If there is any doubt, discuss with GP or the original prescriber.
- Advise the patient when the next injection is due.
- Report any deterioration in the patient's mental state to the GP or secondary care nurse if they are still in contact.
- Make sure there is an injection available for the next appointment.
- Always look out for side effects. Carry out a comprehensive assessment every three months by using a recognised side effect rating score such as SESCAM (see Chapter 9).
- Check the patient has had their physical health check. Arrange if necessary and discuss the benefits with the patient.

Prescribing antipsychotic medicines

The lowest effective dose of antipsychotic medication should be prescribed. Sometimes the patient's symptoms will exacerbate, and require a temporary (weeks to months) increase in their dose of medication. The length of therapy with antipsychotic medication is individual, though most patients with chronic schizophrenia will need to take an antipsychotic for the rest of their lives. Patients who have a good understanding of their illness and are aware that increased symptoms may be a warning sign for relapse, can often manage without medication or with a reduced dose.

The stopping of antipsychotic drugs after long-term therapy should be undertaken by a mental health specialist. It should always be gradual and closely monitored to avoid the risk of acute withdrawal syndrome or rapid relapse.

Medicines used for people with bipolar disorder

Treatment of bipolar disorder is dependent on the patient's phase of illness: acute manic or mixed; acute depressive symptoms; long-term treatment; special treatment considerations (the elderly, women of child bearing age). The choice of treatment should be based on patient preference, evidence of efficacy, side effects, safety and the potential for interactions with other drugs.

Acute or mixed episode

Medication is essential in the treatment of an acute manic or mixed episode of bipolar disorder. Patients may also require admission to hospital or intensive input from a crisis or home treatment team. There is robust evidence that antipsychotic medicines such as olanzapine, quetiapine, risperidone and aripiprazole are highly effective in quickly bringing mania under control (Goodwin, 2009). Potential side effects of these medicines are shown in Table 10.1 (page 85). Psychosis that often accompanies mania is also effectively treated with antipsychotic medication. Valproate is a possible alternative treatment for mania. Lithium (that requires close monitoring, summarised in Table 10.2, page 86) or carbamazapine are also effective anti-manic medicines, but seem to be better suited to patients with less severe mania because it generally seems to take at least a week for these drugs to work. The side effects of valproate, lithium and carbamzapine are summarised in Table 10.3 (page 86).

Sleep problems and behavioural disturbance are common in mania and patients may benefit from PRN benzodiazepines. Antidepressant medication can 'flip' patients with bipolar depression into a manic phase of their illness; it should be gradually stopped in patients experiencing a manic episode of illness. Psychological treatments are not effective in this phase of the illness.

Acute depressive episode

The treatment of bipolar depression is, perhaps, more challenging than that of mania. The medicines that may perhaps first come to mind are antidepressants. Whilst generally SSRIs (the side effects of which are described earlier in this chapter) are generally – though not all researchers agree with this view – considered effective against bipolar depression there is a risk that they can 'flip' patients into mania. Antidepressants that have a dual action such as venlafaxine and older tricyclic medicines seem to be much more likely to provoke a switch into mania and should be avoided in the treatment of bipolar depression. One way of protecting against a switch into mania is to co-prescribe patients lithium, valproate or an antipsychotic. Whilst this is an effective strategy there are considerable disadvantages to this approach; treatment regimes become more complex and medication-related side effects may increase. As there is no compelling evidence that antidepressants in bipolar depression long-term are helpful it is considered good practice after 12 weeks to taper treatment off and stop (Goodwin, 2009).

Lamotrigine may be a potentially helpful treatment for bipolar depression. Evidence of efficacy is far from convincing however and rash is a common side effect. Other common side effects include dizziness, nausea and coordination problems. In patients who have previously experienced switch to mania from antidepressant medication, lamotrigine may be a treatment choice worth considering.

The treatment of choice in bipolar depression is probably quetiapine. There is compelling evidence from a number of randomised controlled trials that both 300mg/day and 600mg/day doses of quetiapine are effective in the treatment of bipolar depression and do not appear to switch patients into mania (Calabrese et al., 2005). There also seems to be additional benefit from quetiapine in the treatment of some of the anxiety symptoms that many bipolar patients experience.

Long-term treatment

Long-term treatment (for at least two years following the first episode of illness) is required in bipolar disorder to prevent the recurrence of both the depressive and manic poles of the illness. Lithium and perhaps valproate and carbamazepine are generally considered as medicines that patients take long-term as a mood stabiliser preventing against relapse to either pole. In truth these medicines seem to be more effective at protecting against one or the other pole but not against both. As a result many bipolar patients will require combination therapy; the consequence is an increased side effect burden and an increased risk of non-adherence.

In no particular order aripiprazole, carbamazepine, lamotrigine, lithium, olanzapine, quetiapine and valproate are effective long-term treatments in bipolar disorder as mono and combination therapies. Quetiapine and valproate are effective in preventing both depression and mania; lithium is more effective against mania than depression and (uniquely) reduces the risk of suicide. Carbamazepine prevents relapse to both poles but is not as effective as lithium. Lamotrigine is more effective against depression than mania. Olanzapine and aripiprazole are effective against mania; olanzapine may also be effective against depression (Goodwin, 2009).

Bipolar disorder and pregnancy

It is not uncommon for patients to become pregnant either by design or accidentally. There are some important considerations when discussing pregnancy in bipolar disorder:

- Medicine used to treat bipolar disorder may affect fertility. For example valproate has been associated with polycystic ovarian syndrome, potentially reducing fertility; carbamazepine on the other hand reduces the effectiveness of the oral contraceptive pill, increasing the risk of unplanned pregnancy.

- There is a known increased risk of major congenital malformations from the medicines used to treat bipolar disorder. For example there is an up to three-fold increase in the risk of malformations in the babies of women taking valproate.

- One in four women will experience a bipolar relapse after childbirth.

Table 10.1 *A rough guide to antipsychotic side effects (adapted from Taylor et al., 2009)*

Antipsychotic	Sedation	Weight gain	Extrapyramidal (movement disorders)	Anti-cholinergic (dry mouth, blurred vision, constipation)	Hypotension	Prolactin elevation (sexual side effects)
Aripiprazole	-	+/-	+/-	-	-	-
Olanzapine	++	+++	+/-	+	++	++
Quetiapine	++	++	-	+	++	+
Risperidone	++	++	+	+	++	+++

Key (incidence/severity): +++ High, ++ moderate, + low, - very low

Table 10.2 *Lithium monitoring*

- Initial dose 400mg at night
- Plasma level seven days after treatment initiated
  Then every seven days until desired level is reached
- Target plasma level in bipolar disorder 0.6–1mmol/L
- Blood should ideally be taken 12 hours after last dose
- Plasma lithium levels every 3 months
- Monitor weight
- e-GFR and TFTs before treatment and then every six months
- Pre-treatment ECG in patients with risk factors for CVD
- Stop slowly over a minimum of 1 month

Table 10.3 *Adverse effects from valproate, lithium and carbamazapine*

Medicine	Adverse effect
Valproate	Nausea, vomiting, sedation, weight gain, ataxia, hair loss (with curly regrowth), peripheral oedema, polycystic ovarian disorder Established risk of teratogenic effects in pregnancy. Should not be used in women of child bearing age
Lithium	Adverse effects directly related to plasma levels ● When levels go above 1 mmol/l: fine hand tremor (propranolol can help), increased thirst, polyuria (more common with twice daily dosing), can make existing acne and psoriasis worse, weight gain ● When levels over 1.5 mmol/l: anorexia, nausea, diarrhoea, muscle weakness, drowsiness, ataxia, coarse tremor, muscle twitching In plasma levels over 2 mmol/l: Disorientation, seizures, coma and death
Carbamazepine	**Frequent**: dizziness, blurred vision, drowsiness, ataxia, nausea **Less frequent**: skin rash, hyponatraemia (low sodium) **Rare**: agranulocytosis, aplastic anaemia, Stevens-Johnson syndrome, pancreatitis

Summary

We have described the appropriate medication for use in depression, anxiety, schizophrenia, bipolar disorder, dementia and sleep disturbance. In some circumstances it may be helpful to liaise with your secondary care colleagues for specific advice.

Gill is 46 years old. She was diagnosed with depression four weeks ago and prescribed citalopram 10mg. She saw the GP two weeks later and reported that she could feel some benefit; the GP increased the dose to 20mg. At her next appointment she reported an increase in sweating. The GP asked if she had any other symptoms. Gill said no and in fact was feeling remarkably better. The GP was satisfied that the sweating was not a symptom of serotonin syndrome and explained that she could continue the citalopram if she could cope with the sweating or another antidepressant could be prescribed. Gill said she felt so much better that she did not really want to stop it. The GP advised her to observe for any other symptoms and report back to him should any new ones occur. He arranged to see her two weeks later.

References

Anderson, I., Nutt, D. and Deakin, J. (2000) Evidence-based guidelines for treating depressive disorders with antidepressants: a revision of the 1993 British Association for Psychopharmacology guidelines. British Association for Psychopharmacology. *Journal of Psychopharmacology* **14**: 3–20.

Calabrese, J., Shelton, M., Rapport, D., Youngstrom, E.A., Jackson, K., Bilali, S., Ganocy, S.J. and Findling, R.L. (2005) A 20 month, double blind, maintenance trial of lithium versus Divalproex in rapid-cycling bipolar disorder. *American Journal of Psychiatry* **162**: 2152–61.

Gill, S.S., Rochon, P.A., Herrmann, N., Lee, P.E., Sykora, K., Gunraj, N., Normand, S-L.T., Gurwitz, J.H., Marras, C., Wodchis, W.P. and Mamdani, M.. (2005) Atypical antipsychotic drugs and risk of ischaemic stroke: population based retrospective cohort study. *British Medical Journal* **76**: 87.

Goodwin, G. (2009) Evidence-based guideline for treating bipolar disorder: revised second edition-recommendations for the British Association for Psychopharmacology. *Journal of Psychopharmacology* **23** (4): 346–88.

Herrmann, N., Mamdani, M. and Lanctot, K. (2004) Atypical antipsychotics and risk of cerebrovascular accidents. *American Journal of Psychiatry* **161**: 1113–15.

McIntyre, R., Muller, A., Mancini, D. and Silver, E.S. (2003) What to do if an initial antidepressant fails? *Canadian Family Physician* **49**: 449–57.

Rapaport, M., Nierenberg, A., Howland, R., Dording, C., Schettler, P.J. and Mischoulon, D. (2011) The treatment of minor depression with St. John's Wort or citalopram: failure to show benefit over placebo. *Journal of Psychiatric Research* **45** (7): 931–41.

Schneider, L., Dagerman, K. and Insel, P. (2005). Risk of death with atypical antipsychotic drug treatment for dementia. *Journal of the American Medical Association* **294**: 1934–43.

Taylor, D., Paton, C. and Kapur S. (2009) *The Maudsley Prescribing Guidelines* 10th Edition. London: Informa Healthcare.

Chapter 11

Other mental health problems

In this chapter we will consider other mental health problems – alcohol misuse, substance abuse, bereavement, and eating disorders – which present in primary care and generally require referral to specialist psychiatric services.

Alcohol misuse

Problem drinking can be divided into alcohol misuse or dependence. Alcohol use is measured in units, one unit equates to half a standard glass or 175ml of wine (alcohol by volume – ABV 12 per cent) or a third of a pint of beer (ABV 5–6 per cent). Misuse is defined as the consumption of over 28 units per week for men, 21 units for women and is associated with an increased risk of physical health problems, for example, liver disease or gastrointestinal bleeding, and psychological health problems, such as depression or anxiety. Alcohol misuse is also associated with negative social consequences (e.g. loss of job).

Alcohol dependence is defined by the presence of three or more of the following:

- a strong craving to use alcohol
- trouble in controlling alcohol use
- withdrawal (anxiety, tremors, sweating) when drinking is stopped
- tolerance (able to drink large amounts of alcohol without becoming drunk)
- continual alcohol use despite damaging consequences.

The consequences of alcohol dependence are considerable and include CVD and stroke.

Raised levels of Gamma Glutamyl Transferase (GGT) and Mean Corpuscular Volume (MCV) are markers that will help identify heavy drinking.

Identifying alcohol problems

Few patients will present saying that they have a drink problem. Most will either deny or be unaware of the seriousness of their alcohol problems. Often coming to light during routine consultations, it is important to be proactive in checking how much alcohol patients are drinking. Some patients present with physical symptoms which are the complications of alcohol use such as ulcer, gastritis, liver disease, accidental injury. A low mood, poor memory or concentration and insomnia may also be a sign that the patient has a problem with alcohol. Problems with alcohol may also come to light when the patients have tried to cut down or stop drinking alcohol and experience withdrawal symptoms that include sweating and tremors.

Alcohol use: cause or effect

Patients may drink to self-medicate an underlying mental health problem, particularly depression. In patients that you identify as misusing or being dependent on alcohol, you should screen for depression (using for example the PHQ-9) and treat appropriately (see Chapter 2).

Treatment of alcohol dependence

Quitting alcohol is tough; many patients will try and lapse several times before they are successful in quitting (or reducing). Trying to scare people to stop drinking by telling them 'if they don't they will die' whilst intuitive is not actually very effective. Helping to reduce or stop alcohol may be more successful with specialist support. In those patients with very serious alcohol dependence and that require detoxification, support from practitioners with appropriate competence will be necessary. Many areas have their own local centre which specialises in helping patients with alcohol problems. Entering the name of your town or postcode into FRANK will enable you to access this information: **http://www.talktofrank.com** (last accessed: 3.1.12). Patients may also find national help lines a useful source of information and advice:

- Alcoholics Anonymous – their helpline number is 0845 769 7555.
- Alcohol Concern run a national drink helpline called 'Drinkline';
  their number is 0800 917 8282.

Quitting or harm reduction

Some patients will not be willing to stop drinking. Harm reduction – encouraging the patient to cut down the amount they drink – may be a helpful step towards quitting. Providing information about the harmful effects of drinking is important. Many patients who abuse alcohol are malnourished resulting in a lack of thiamine (vitamin B1) which helps maintain the functioning of the heart and nervous and digestive systems. Reducing alcohol can precipitate acute loss of thiamine stores in patients who are already chronically thiamine deficient. Thiamine deficiency is associated with Wernicke-Korsakoff syndrome (alcoholic brain disease) and beriberi (neurological symptoms, cardiovascular abnormalities and oedema). It may be worth considering a thiamine preparation to prevent these conditions.

Drug misuse

Cannabis, cocaine, heroin, speed and ecstasy are examples of drugs of misuse. Identification of drug misuse is difficult; many patients will deny that they have a problem and in any case it is rare for primary care practitioners to proactively screen patients for substance use. There are some patients who use non-prescription drugs to self-medicate an underlying mental health problem. Typically drug misuse will come to light when the patient presents at the surgery in a distressed state requesting help. In our experience patients want:

- a prescription for drugs
- help to withdraw or stabilise their drug use
- treatment for the physical complications of drug use, such as abscesses
- medical acknowledgement of a drug problem because of debt or prosecution.

Diagnosis

The diagnosis of a substance misuse disorder should be based on a comprehensive history. We suggest you ask the following questions:

- Has using drugs resulted in:
  - physical injury or illness?
  - emotional distress or mental illness?
  - social problems such as breakdown of relationships, job loss?
- How often do you take drugs?
- In a typical week how much alcohol do you drink?

- Do you crave drugs?
- Are you unable to stop using drugs?
- Do the drugs you take no longer have the effect they used to?
- Do you have withdrawal symptoms when you stop taking drugs (increased heart rate, sweating, tremors)?
- What are your reasons for attending the surgery today?
- Have you got a past history of physical or mental illness?

Your examination of the patient should include:

- checking for physical symptoms e.g. nausea, constipation, drowsiness;
- screening for depression using the PHQ-9 (Chapter 2);
- laboratory investigations, specifically a full blood count, liver function test, hepatitis B and C screen, urine drug screen.

The advice you give will be dependent on whether the patient wants to continue using drugs or consider stopping. You should pass no judgement if they wish to continue but offer advice about the benefits of stopping (improved physical and mental health, ability to sort out social problems). You should offer referral to your local NHS drug misuse service or advise them of self-help organisations. These include:

- CITAP (Council for Involuntary Tranquilliser Addiction, and Painkillers) 0151 932 0102.
- Narcotics Anonymous 0300 999 1212.
- Release 0845 450 0215.

Bereavement

Grief is a common and normal reaction to the death of someone close or following a major life event such as the breakdown of relationship or redundancy. It is important to remember that grief, although difficult and distressing, is a process that most people will work through without the need for treatment. There are usually four stages to the grief process:

- accepting the loss
- feeling the pain
- becoming accustomed to the loss
- letting go and moving on.

People who are working through the grief process will often be emotional; they may be frequently sad and tearful, angry, disbelieving of what has happened, anxious and irritable or guilty. Preoccupation and thinking that they have seen or heard the person who has died are common. Quite naturally people will want to talk, seemingly constantly, about what has happened to them.

Some patients do not naturally work their way through this process and get stuck, sometimes for many years. For others bereavement can exacerbate existing mental health problems and in some patients psychiatric conditions, particularly depression, can be triggered by the stress caused by a loss. These groups of patients may benefit from treatment.

Depression is perhaps the most common mental health problem associated with bereavement and seems to be more common if:

- the patient is socially isolated
- the patient was having relationship problems with the person who died
- it was a traumatic or violent death, for example in a car crash, murder or suicide
- the person who died was young
- no body was found.

What you can do:

- Provide an opportunity for the patient to talk about the person who died and the circumstances of the death.
- Ask the patient about their feelings regarding the loss.
- Explain that it will take time for them to come to terms with their loss and that the emotional pain should fade over the coming months.
- Advise them to take time out if needed (break from work, reduce other commitments).
- Monitor the patient's mood, checking for symptoms of depression:
  - Treat any emergent depressive disorder appropriately (see Chapter 2).
  - Refer the patient for (bereavement) counselling if they are not progressing through the grief process:
    Compassionate Friends 0845 123 2304 (for bereaved parents, siblings and grandparents)
    Cruse Bereavement Care 0844 477 9400 (one-to-one bereavement counselling)

Papyrus 0800 068 4141 (for parents of young people who have committed suicide)

Still Birth and Neonatal Death Society (SANDS) 020 7436 5881 (for parents who have lost a baby).

Eating disorders

Although there are a number of eating disorders, the two most common are anorexia and bulimia. Patients with either condition may come and see you with a physical complaint such as palpitations, amenorrhoea and even fits. Often it is a parent or close family member who will come to see you or persuade the patient to come in as they are concerned about their refusal to eat, loss of weight or vomiting.

The characteristics of both conditions may be:

- an irrational fear of gaining weight
- denial that their eating habits are abnormal
- working excessively to prevent weight gain, for example vomiting, restricting food, laxative use, extreme exercising
- becoming withdrawn
- relationship problems
- work or school difficulties
- obsessional behaviour
- irritability or low mood.

Some patients may display both anorexic and bulimic characteristics on different occasions.

The specific characteristics of anorexia nervosa are:

- belief that they are overweight (distorted body image)
- strict dieting, despite very low weight (body mass index <17.5 kg/m2)
- amenorrhoea.

The specific characteristics of bulimia are:

- binge-eating (eating huge amounts of food in a short space of time)
- purging (trying to get rid of food by vomiting or by using diuretics or laxatives).

Complications caused by eating disorders

- Severe weight loss can cause amenorrhea, dental problems, muscle weakness, renal stones, constipation and liver dysfunction.
- Purging can cause dental problems, salivary-gland swelling, renal stones, cardiac arrhythmias and fits.

Management of eating disorders

We suggest you establish a regular routine of attendance and:

- Perform a risk assessment:
  - Features of high medical risk include excess exercise with low weight, blood in vomit, inadequate fluid intake and poor nutrition, rapid weight loss and factors that disrupt ritualised eating behaviours (travelling/exams).
- Provide education about a healthy diet and weight.
- Refer to dietician if this service is available.
- Ask what the benefits and disadvantages of the condition are for the patient and discuss.
- Monitor weight, setting realistic targets agreed with the patient.
- Advise about local voluntary or self-help groups.

Treatment

Anorexia

Treatment should be matched against patient need and based on a careful risk assessment of medical, clinical and psychosocial factors. There is no evidence to suggest medication will be helpful unless there is an underlying condition such as depression. Consider family psychotherapy if the patient is under 18 years of age or individual psychotherapy for an adult.

Bulimia

To avoid binging, encourage the patient to eat regular meals; using a meal planner and food diary may be helpful to achieve this. Discuss what alternative activity can be undertaken when the patient feels the urge to binge, for example, go for a walk, telephone a friend, play a computer game.

Fluoxetine (60mg/day) can be an effective treatment. CBT may be helpful. This can be accessed through your IAPT service.

When should you refer to secondary mental health services with expertise in eating disorders?

You should make an urgent referral if:

- there is a high risk of suicide
- body mass index is <13.5
- potassium levels are <2.5 mmol/l
- platelet levels are low
- there is severe muscle atrophy and weakness
- there are major gastrointestinal symptoms from repeated vomiting
- there are other complications such as alcohol or substance abuse.

You should make a routine referral if your patient is not progressing.

National organisations that are a useful resource in treating eating disorders are:

National Centre for Eating Disorders **http://www.eating-disorders.org.uk/** (last accessed 3.1.12).

Beating Eating Disorders (BEAT) **http://www.b-eat.co.uk/** (last accessed 3.1.12).

Summary

We have briefly described four conditions (alcohol misuse, drug misuse, bereavement and eating disorders) commonly seen in primary care but which would ideally benefit from specialist intervention. In practice you may find that you are left with the responsibility of managing their care. We urge you to seek advice and guidance from the sources that we have listed to assist you in providing effective care and treatment.

Case Study

David is 48 years old. He has diabetes and regularly sees the practice nurse for check ups. He explains to her that sometimes he feels light headed and faint and wondered if it was his diabetes. She said it certainly sounded like it could be low blood glucose. She checked his last average blood glucose reading and it was raised (IFCC-HbA1c 100mmol/mol) and the medication he was taking (metformin) does not cause hypoglycaemia (low blood glucose). She explained this to David who asked what else could cause low blood glucose in diabetes. She answered either vigorous exercise or alcohol. David then admitted that he had been dependent on alcohol for a long time and was drinking eight cans of Special Brew a day.

The practice nurse asked David if he wanted to change this. He said he had been to the local drug and alcohol centre before and did not want to go back. He explained that he would like to try to reduce his alcohol consumption and asked if the practice nurse would help. The practice nurse advised him she was not an expert in this field but would be happy to assist. She recommended that he had blood tests and saw the doctor who may prescribe medication. David agreed.

Chapter 12

A rough guide to the Mental Health Act

Some patients, when severely mentally unwell, may need to be detained in hospital under mental health law. Generally patients are detained because their health is threatened or there is a serious risk of harm to themselves or others. England and Scotland have different mental health legislation. Information on English law can be found at **http://www.legislation.gov.uk/ukpga/2007/12/contents** (last accessed 23.1.12) and Scottish law at **http://www.scotland.gov.uk/Topics/Health/health/mental-health/mhlaw** (last accessed 3.1.12). Primary care practitioners are most likely to need to resort to mental health law if a seriously unwell patient in the surgery or community is refusing to go to secondary care and they are concerned about the level of risk they present. On occasions GPs will be called (normally by the patient's family or friends or community mental health workers) to the patient's home because they are seriously mentally unwell and may require compulsory admission and treatment. In England the detention of a patient will generally require the opinion of at least one doctor and an approved mental health professional (AMHP – a mental health nurse or social worker).

The parts of the Act that you probably need to be aware of are:

- Section 4 – A maximum 72-hour emergency admission for assessment enacted by a doctor and an AMHP.
- Section 136 – This section allows a police officer to remove a patient at risk to a place of safety. It lasts up to 72 hours and permits the patient to be assessed by a medical practitioner.
- Section 2 – A maximum 28-day admission for assessment enacted by two doctors and an AMHP.
- Section 3 – A maximum six-month admission for treatment enacted by two

doctors and an AMHP. The nearest relative must give their consent. This section can be renewed if further treatment is necessary.

Community Treatment Orders (CTOs) in England were introduced in 2007 as part of the amendment to the 1983 Mental Health Act. Requiring patients to take medication whilst in the community under threat of recall to hospital if they are non-adherent, CTOs have proved surprisingly popular. It is perhaps worth noting that there is little evidence to demonstrate that CTOs are effective in ensuring that patients adhere to treatment.

Summary

Compulsory treatment of mental illness is a last resort. That said, leaving patients unwell and untreated will do irreversible harm. Judiciously applied mental health law is an important and necessary element in the treatment of mental illness.

Case Study

Martin is 19 years old and has had no previous contact with mental health services. His mother called the GP because Martin had not come out of his bedroom for two weeks other than to use the toilet. He had a supply of biscuits, crisps and fizzy drinks but no other food. In the last two days he had begun to shout abuse from the window to passers-by. When his mother had tried to talk to him he swore and told her to leave him alone making accusations that she was out to hurt him. On this particular day, Martin had thrown a bottle out of the window aimed at an elderly neighbour. Fortunately it missed. The GP considered contacting the mental health services to initiate admission under Section 4 of the Mental Health Act. However, as they would be unable to gain access to Martin he contacted the police to take Martin to a place of safety where he could be assessed by a medical practitioner under Section 136.

Index